CHILDREN WITH ASTHMA
A Manual for Parents

by

THOMAS F. PLAUT, M.D.

With Parents, Patients and Physicians

Pedipress
Amherst, Massachusetts

NOTICE

The indications and dosages of all drugs in this book have been recommended in the medical literature and conform to the practices of the general medical community. The medications described do not necessarily have specific approval by the Food and Drug Administration for use in the ages and dosages and indications for which they are recommended. The package insert for each drug should be consulted for use and dosage as approved by the FDA. Because standards for usage change, it is advisable to keep abreast of revised recommendations. <u>Consult your physician before making any change in medication.</u>

Library of Congress Cataloging in Publication Data

    Plaut, Thomas F.
      Children with asthma

1. Asthma in children. I. Title. [DNLM: 1. Asthma --In infancy and childhood--Popular works. WF 553 P721c] RJ436. A8P56 1983   618.92'238   83-19444

ISBN 0914625-02-0

First printing 1983
Second printing 1984 revised
Third printing 1985
Fourth printing 1987

Copyright 1984, 1983 Thomas F. Plaut.
All rights reserved. No part of the book may be reproduced in any form or by any electronic or mechanical means, including information storage and retrieval systems without permission in writing from the publisher, except by a reviewer who may quote brief passages in a review.

Published by Pedipress, Inc., 125 Red Gate Lane, Amherst, MA 01002.
Printed in the United States of America.

Dedicated to parents, patients and physicians
who are willing to learn.

ABOUT THE AUTHOR

Thomas F. Plaut, M.D. has practiced pediatrics for twenty years. With his three pediatric colleagues, he cares for more than four hundred children with asthma. Plaut became interested in asthma education nine years ago when he had trouble finding information adequate to answer the questions of his patients.

He read extensively about asthma and then asked experts across the country to clarify controversial points. Patients made an equally important contribution. They asked difficult questions and demanded understandable answers. They observed their children's daily reaction to asthma and the medications used to treat it. They taught their pediatrician about aspects of asthma that he could never observe in the office.

Plaut grew up in Ohio, graduated from Yale University with a degree in history and received his medical degree from Columbia University. After a pediatric residency at New York University-Bellevue Medical Center in New York City, he practiced in Whitesburg, Kentucky and then spent ten years at the Martin Luther King Health Center in the South Bronx. He joined Amherst Medical Associates in 1977.

Plaut believes that almost every parent whose child has asthma has the ability and the desire to learn to manage asthma at home. Most health professionals grossly underestimate this ability. He believes that hospitalization for asthma should be rare. Only six patients from his practice were hospitalized for asthma in 1985.

The author has presented his views on asthma to parents, teachers, and the general public at lectures, seminars, and on radio and television. He regularly offers workshops and presents his research findings to health professionals at local and national meetings.

NOTES ON THE 1984 REVISED EDITION

CHILDREN WITH ASTHMA has been enthusiastically received by parents and health professionals across the country.

This second printing gives me the opportunity to cover several changes that are taking place in the treatment of asthma.

- Cromolyn is being used more frequently as a first-line drug in children who need daily medication.

- Inhaled beta-adrenergics can now be used effectively by many children ages three and over with the aid of a reservoir.

- Infants with asthma can often be kept out of the hospital by using a powered nebulizer to deliver beta-adrenergic drugs and/or cromolyn at home.

New accounts by parents have been added:

"Casey" tells how a mother learned to control her son's asthma. "Knowledge of asthma is the best gift anyone has ever given me."

"Michelle and the Bubble" recounts the use of a bubble reservoir by a three-year-old.

"Nathan" portrays asthma in infancy. He was hospitalized four times in five months but not once in the two years since he started an aggressive treatment program.

Credits:

Chapter 2, page 36. Top illustration and Chapter 3, page 56, "Overview of Medication," adapted from "Manual for Children: Self-Management of Asthma" by Backiel M., Creer T., Leung P. Copyright 1980. Used by permission of T. Creer

Chapter 2, page 36. Middle illustration adapted from Teaching Myself About Asthma. Parcel G., Tiernan K., Nader P., and Weiner L., with illustrations by Mark Weakley. Copyright Guy Parcel. Used by permission of Guy Parcel.

ACKNOWLEDGEMENTS

Parents of children with asthma at Amherst Medical Associates have been involved in every step of this book's development. They asked for basic information that was not available in an appropriate form for parents. They learned about asthma and felt strongly that other parents should be spared the misinformation, inadequate treatment and lack of support with which they had to contend. Jeamie Duffy sat down one night, and after writing for six hours, completed "Matthew," the account of her son's first seven years. Reading that account encouraged other parents to write of their experiences. Harriet Cohen, Dana Parker, Gail Hall and Joe Duffy all tell different stories but the message is the same. You can manage your child's asthma at home if you attain a certain level of knowledge and skills, have a positive attitude and the support of your physician.

Other contributors include Kathy Bowler, Cecelia Cobbs, Celine Cyran, Monica Cyran, Reneé Cyran, Joan Platz, David Plaut and Sherry Polito. None of them are professional writers but their words convey the thoughts of parents and teenagers each of whom have a different angle on the problems of children with asthma.

The entire pediatric staff at Amherst Medical Associates contributed to the production of this book by treating our patients with competence, caring and respect. I want to single out Edna McAveney, Lois Kelley, R.N., Mary Dent, R.N., Linda Haney, R.N., Rosemary Kofler, R.N., Cathy Boyd, R.N., and Leslie Champoux. Michael Posner, M.D. wrote "Coughing Asthma." Sharon Dorfman, health educator, helped me design the first parent's group and made me realize that parents need more than facts and skills.

Kathleen Morrissey drew the illustrations. Caitlin Whittle, word processor, provided diligent help and friendly suggestions.

Thomas Creer, Ph.D., Chairman, Department of Psychology, Ohio University, and Guy Parcel, Ph.D., Director, Division of Health Education, University of Texas Medical Branch, Galveston, Texas, were generous in providing information and encouragement throughout this entire project. Robert Zwerdling, M.D., pediatric pulmonologist, University of Massachusetts Medical School, Worcester, made helpful suggestions. Paul Walker, M.D., allergist, Springfield, Massachusetts, has helped me sort out difficult aspects of asthma, both for my practice and the book.

Emlen Jones, M.D., my partner at AMA, developed several of the handouts and helped refine others. He has been responsible for initiating many of the changes we have made in the treatment of children with asthma over the past five years. His cooperation was essential to this project. I want to recognize him here as an excellent clinician and a hardworking and thoughtful colleague.

Finally I want to thank David for discussing asthma with me, Rebecca for her help with typing and my wife Johanna for her editing. Thanks to the three of you for tolerating the disruption which this book caused in our family's life.

ACKNOWLEDGEMENTS 1984-85

New contributors are Lynn Arseneau, Marilyn Sansouci, and Caroline Tropp.

The pediatric staff at Amherst Medical Associates are all involved in the care of our patients with asthma. Beth Coxon, Sally Howland, R.N., Mary Wing, R.N., Martha Barstow, R.N., Anne Gray, Norma Hallock, P.N.P., Ruth Sullivan, P.N.P., Diana Kocot, and Lori Kolasinski have enabled us to increase the service we provide to patients.

Over the past year several experts have helped me sort out new information on asthma. Miles Weinberger, M.D., Professor of Pediatrics, University of Iowa, Jay Selcow, M.D., Hartford, Connecticut, Carlton Palm, M.D., New Haven, Connecticut, Gregory Fritz, M.D., Palo Alto, California, and Guillermo Mendoza, M.D., Los Angeles, California each provided useful insights.

My three pediatric colleagues, Emlen Jones, M.D., Arlen Collins, M.D., David Marsh, M.D. and I share in the treatment of all children with asthma at Amherst Medical Associates. Their thoughtful observations continue to improve our ability to diagnose and treat children with asthma.

Cover collaborators: David Must, Michael Cohen, and Norman Newell.

TABLE OF CONTENTS

INTRODUCTION

Childhood asthma is a chronic illness that affects about five percent of the children in the United States. It is frequently undertreated and causes more hospital admissions, more visits to hospital emergency rooms and more school absences than any other chronic disease of childhood. Because of its unpredictability, asthma disrupts the living patterns of the children affected by it.

A child may experience an attack suddenly with little warning, causing panic and upheaval in the family unprepared to deal with it. His parents may worry incessantly and needlessly about his well-being. When an asthma attack occurs in school, it causes anxiety for everyone around: the child, the teacher and the nurse. Attacks also interfere with extra-curricular activities. An attack during a sporting event embarrasses the child with asthma and often brings advice to reduce activity. Such restrictions damage the child's self-esteem and are usually unnecessary.

Can we improve the ability of parents and their children with asthma to manage asthma at home? The answer is a definite yes.

We care for 8000 children in our practice; four hundred of them have asthma. We have used existing educational materials and have developed our own to teach parents how to manage asthma at home. Our patients with asthma generally lead normal lives. We enable parents to gain the knowledge, skill, and attitude essential to manage an attack of asthma at home. They learn the pathophysiology of asthma and how medications work. They become proficient in assessing the severity of an attack, keeping an asthma diary and using an inhaler and a peak flow meter. They develop an attitude of autonomy, ready and able to manage most acute attacks of asthma, consulting us if they need help.

Ten years ago, there was no satisfactory way to control asthma in a child with mild to moderate disease. The best a parent could do was to give a combination medication for a mild attack and to bring the child to the doctor's office or emergency room for a shot of adrenalin in the case of a more severe episode.

Recently, several changes have occurred which can render asthma a much more manageable illness:
- theophylline has been recognized as the first-line medication for asthma.
- a test to measure the blood level of theophylline has been developed and is now readily available. This helps us

determine whether the theophylline is at a level that is both effective and safe.

- long-acting preparations of theophylline have been developed. Since they require less frequent administration and cause fewer side effects, their use leads to improved compliance.
- the use of beta-adrenergic drugs by inhaler, in disrepute in the 1970's, is now better understood and can provide a great benefit to many patients.
- new delivery systems (extenders and powered nebulizers) have made inhaled beta adrenergic drugs available to all children with asthma.
- cromolyn sodium has proved to be effective in preventing attacks in many children who have chronic asthma.
- a greater interest in self-care by many Americans has provided a climate in which parents are willing to learn how to play a significant role in managing their child's asthma.
- an inexpensive peak flow meter has been developed. It measures the flow of air from the lung. Physicians can use it in the office to measure progress in treating an attack. Used at home, it can aid in regulating medication and predicting attacks.

Each of these advances provides a significant margin of improvement for many children with asthma. As a group, they are truly powerful. A well-informed parent who understands the management of asthma can now make reliable judgments about the child's situation. The parent can control most attacks without panic and without consulting a physician. The child with moderate asthma can now lead a normal life, taking part in all sports and social activities.

Chapter One
LIVING WITH ASTHMA

Casey's mom writes "Knowledge of asthma is the best gift anyone has ever given me." Harriet Cohen describes Josh's early symptoms, her dealings with doctors and teachers and her learning about asthma over a ten-year period. Dana Parker captures the physical and emotional trauma of a first attack of asthma and tells how his family deals with attacks now. Jeamie Duffy chronicles the first seven years in her son Matthew's life. We learn of the reactions of neighbors and friends and her own evolution from asthma-obsessed mother to a parent with appropriate concerns. Nathan was hospitalized four times in five months but not once in the two years since he started an aggressive treatment program.

CASEY

By Caroline Tropp

Casey was approximately fifteen months old when he was diagnosed as having asthma. It started as a cold, then grew much worse. We brought him to a pediatrician who gave him an injection of adrenalin and some medicine by mouth. Because I hadn't known anyone with asthma, I had no idea of the severity of his problem. I didn't know what his illness would entail and how it would affect our future. Casey's doctor told me to give him medicine, which seemed to make him better. Casey took it for a few days and he was fine. A week or two after I stopped the medicine he started wheezing, coughing and moaning--just like the first time. It was then that I realized that asthma would affect not only Casey, but the whole family.

Every time Casey would have an attack (usually in the middle of the night) we would take him to the emergency room and pray that they could bring his attack under control. Usually we would bring him home. Three times the attack was so severe that he was admitted to the hospital for a few days. If you've ever had a child in the hospital, you know the pain and helpless feelings that you go through. When they tell you to go home and your baby is screaming for you to stay, it tears your heart out to leave him there.

Well, all this went on for about two years. It seemed that as soon as Casey started to get a cold or the flu, it would bring on an asthma attack. We would give him his medicine and pray. He often ended up in the hospital emergency room. It put a strain on all of us. We didn't understand why our beautiful baby boy had such a severe problem. We felt so helpless. I think you blame yourself for not being able to help your child at his time of need. When friends or relatives would phone, their first question would be, "How's Casey's asthma?" I was so frustrated about the whole situation that I remember just crying when he would start wheezing because I knew what would be in store for us. The thing that sticks out most in my mind is that the doctors would say that he would probably grow out of it. Big deal! Was that supposed to help me now?

Casey was almost three years old when we had to switch doctors because of a change in my health insurance. I called to see the new doctor about Casey because I wanted him to become familiar with Casey before he had another attack. I was really surprised when the receptionist said that one of the pediatricians was an asthma specialist. I thought to myself maybe we had found someone who could help my little boy.

When we arrived at the office I was hoping that he could help me. But I kept thinking maybe he, like the others, would just say, "Casey will probably grow out of his asthma." The pediatrician came into the examining room and introduced himself. He started asking me questions about the medication Casey was taking. Well, he wasn't taking any one medication. I had about eight medicines in the house in case of an attack. I couldn't remember half their names, not to mention what they would do for my child. I felt so dumb because all I knew was that my child had asthma. I knew nothing about the causes of his asthma attacks or about possible side-effects or correct doses of his medications.

After the pediatrician reviewed the full story of Casey's asthma with me he examined Casey from head to toe. Then we sent Casey to play in the waiting room while we talked. The doctor started by saying "Casey has moderately severe asthma but we will probably be able to prevent him from staying in the hospital again." We (the doctor and I) would be a team in combatting his illness. He prescribed medications and explained them fully. Casey would be on medication constantly now. We sat for approximately half an hour and discussed Casey and what I had to know about treating him at home. I thought I had finally found someone who could help us. I had been in the dark for so long and was finally seeing the light at the end of the tunnel. Why did the other doctors assume that they were the only ones capable of treating and understanding my child with asthma? Why couldn't I learn? Why wouldn't they take the time to teach me? All the heartache of Casey's illness could have been minimized years ago.

Do you know, my new doctor never mentioned the fact that Casey might grow out of it? His concern is treating him NOW! Casey is doing exceptionally well now. He takes medication daily and has some backup medication. I finally feel that everything is under control. He has had a few attacks, but I now know how to treat him at home with much success. I feel like I'm in the driver's seat finally after all these years. My doctor is just a phone call away if I need him. Knowledge and understanding of this illness is the best gift anyone has ever given me.

JOSH

By Harriet Cohen

"How long has this baby been wheezing?" asked the pediatrician in Peterborough, New Hampshire, for whose arrival we had all been praying as the few g.p.'s were so overworked already. He didn't ask this question politely. There was a nasty, guilt-producing edge to the question. Like, "Lady, how long have you been so dumb?" In truth, I had brought eighteen-month old Josh in because he had had this odd, sharp cough all morning. There didn't seem to be any cold symptoms. I was torn between ignoring it and taking him in, thereby running the risk of being laughed at as an over-anxious mother. Minor anxiety won out over self-image. I'll just get this checked out, thought I.

"What's wheezing?" I asked. And that was how I learned that my second and heretofore perfectly normal, (well, almost) healthy baby had asthma (italics mine) -- What a curse! Everyone knew asthma was a psychosomatic disease caused, of course, by mother! Oh God, Sigmund Freud has my number. This is it. I thought I had been doing such a good job of faking parenting.

Now came the shot of adrenalin. Then the twenty-minute wait in the waiting room while he turned ghastly pale white. Then the slightly congratulatory welcome back to the second shot--well good, adrenalin will work on him. And then the prescription for a combination theophylline preparation (asthma syrup), to be administered every few hours for the next few days and then, after that, as needed. There was probably a followup visit. It's hard to remember. Josh is now almost twelve. He was born in 1970. So this story starts about nine and a half years ago.

Looking back, one can pick out a few minor hints that something odd might be in store for Josh. I brought him home from the hospital in little gauze booties that the nurses had made for his feet, and gauze mitts for his hands. Apparently he was allergic to detergents in the hospital sheets and his fingers and toes were raw and bleeding until the nurses took pity and improvised protection. His sister, two years older, had eczema; Josh had it too, but not as severely. Later, when the doctors began to look at the allergy histories in our family, I discovered that a baby my mother had before me had died of "milk poisoning" while being treated in New York for extremely severe eczema at the age of eight months. The "milk poisoning" was deduced by the allergist to have probably been an allergic reaction to milk. At eight months, just as I weaned him from the breast, Josh too became allergic to milk. I was advised to try soy-milk formula but he vomited that up. The Peterborough pediatrician was thoroughly mystified. He said, well, just skip milk. This worried me so much that I cajoled him into giving me some calcium pills. I have always worried that the month or two that passed without milk at that critical growth period may have somehow affected Josh for life.

We got Josh back on milk by offering him ice cream a few months later. When he seemed to tolerate it, we tried milk and the problem was over. Not until Josh was three did we determine that he was allergic to peanuts. When we moved to Amherst, the new pediatrician advised us to have a complete allergy run-down because of this, and also because Josh was congested and wheezy on and off. We were told to ask the allergist if there was any serum to help develop resistance to the peanut allergy or whether Josh would outgrow it. The symptoms were severe vomiting, followed by an asthma attack which we treated as best we could with the asthma syrup. A visit to the Springfield allergist revealed that he was, indeed, in the very highest category of allergy to peanuts (and soy beans, lentils, legumes in general) and very serious warnings ensued, along with a prescription for a bee-sting kit. No other serious allergies showed up; there was a minor allergy to dogs. Big sister was allergic to cats, so there were no pets at home. One of Josh's worst asthma attacks during this period followed a weekend visit to friends with an adorable puppy.

The years between Josh at three, with "occasional" asthma and Josh at seven, when what I can only describe as our "awakening" (to the true nature of his condition) occurred, are something of a blur to me. Josh was always runny-nosed. I don't remember using asthma syrup very often. Once in the middle of the night, he seemed to be having difficulty. I called the pediatrician. He recommended that we put Josh in the car and roll down the window and take him for a ride in the icy winter air (which we could not bring ourselves to do).

Yet there must have been some attention paid to his condition. I do remember a bout of several months where we tried cromolyn capsules. There was no way that this five (or four, or six ??) year old could master the tricky technique involved. Half the dust blew out of the capsule and into the air. Maybe a smidge went into his lungs. I drove a fourteen mile round trip to save five dollars on every prescription renewal. After a while I guess we just gave up on cromolyn. Maybe the doctor let us off the hook. Maybe Josh's intermittent wheezing wasn't helped. In those days I was so oblivious and ignorant. I remember worrying a lot more about peanuts and about Josh's inability to perform in school.

When he went to private kindergarten at age five, they called and told me that he seemed more comfortable with the "fours" and seemed to belong there. That was fine with me, as I could tell that he was nowhere near ready to deal even with the pre-reading. He was quite small for his age as well. The constant runny nose made him seem a bit sickly, along with his small, skinny size, I guess.

In the first grade he had a beginning, inexperienced teacher. She seemed not to worry about Josh's continuing inability to deal with reading and writing. She said he often appeared tired and would nap under her desk during the afternoon. Perhaps his constant runny nose wasn't helping things either? He was immature for his age, but not to worry. Boys often are small and immature, and usually they begin to grow up and to read at the same time, and it is too early to worry in the first grade. That's what she said. What I saw was a child who wished he didn't have to go to school--who begged to stay home as the second grade began.

The second grade teacher, a woman with a great deal of experience and warmth, was on the phone after a month and a half. A core evaluation was prescribed. Josh was diagnosed as chronically depressed by a school psychiatric consultant. He was also unable to work in a large group or small remedial group situation. He had learned virtually nothing in a year and a half of school. He was beginning to get into fights with other students. This evaluation procedure dragged on for a long time. Finally, the school said it would pay for a psychiatrist to see Josh. I remember clearly that it was already April, and both the one-to-one special tutor they hired for Josh and the friendly "guidance counselor" who worked with him were at their wits' end.

The day we took him to see the psychiatrist for the first time this doctor commented to us that Josh seemed very unwell. We agreed and said that perhaps April was a poor month for Josh allergy-wise. That night, Josh had his first really severe asthma attack in a long time. I don't remember taking him in for adrenalin hardly at all in the four years that we had been in Amherst. But that night, we were told to bring him in, instead of driving him around the block. There we met the new pediatrician, who had recently taken over from the previous practitioner. In between the first shot and the second one, he grilled us. What were we doing for this child's wheezing? I felt again that guilty pang that I had felt in Peterborough.

The doctor seemed astounded and appalled when I told him that I gave Josh medication only if I heard him wheeze. "You've got to continue medication for at least two days after wheezing stops," he said. Well, I was pretty well recovered from my Adele Davis period, but those words were bitter pills to swallow still (no pun intended). Patiently he explained that he, too, was reluctant to prescribe unless absolutely necessary. But, he insisted, asthma must be dealt with from the approach of using the medication as prophylaxis. Medicine as prevention. Medicine constantly around the clock, day-in and day-out. My little boy had asthma.

It was as if I had never heard the words before. Deep shock set in. I had a very close friend who suffered terribly from asthma. His grandmother had died from it. His own mother lived on steroids. His life was a ritual of pills, steroids, antacid to fight the side effects of the steroids, and trying to stay up until one or two in the morning so as not to miss a dose. Trying not to use the inhaler. Using the inhaler. Hiding from smoke-filled parties, unable to dance in smoky rooms. Spending a good percentage of his small income on all the different medicines he needed to stay alive. This friend used to tell me that Josh was wheezing. I would bring Josh to swim at his lake cottage and he would say, "Harriet, Josh is wheezing." "Oh, its nothing," I would say. At this time, Josh was four or five years old. Not my Josh, he didn't have asthma. Not like that. And again, my friend dropped over, saw Josh, and said warningly, "He's wheeeeeeezing." He tried to help Josh master the cromolyn inhaler which he used himself. Why hadn't I taken it more seriously? I will never know. Perhaps just ignorance. I do know that it wasn't just Josh who had to be treated. I, we (Josh's father and I) now had to be educated right along with Josh.

The first revelation was about the asthma syrup. Combination medicines are no longer recommended by the experts said Josh's doctor. They contain unnecessary ingredients which can lead to bad side effects. So it was out with the combo and in with theophylline. We had one phyllin, this phyllin and that phyllin. At last, we settled on a long-acting theophylline tablet and taught Josh to master the fine art of pill-swallowing. What a breakthrough that was! Liberation from pouring liquids into those plastic measuring vial-spons, and dribbling it down the poor child's throat. All this while, the pediatrician held our hands (Mike's and mine, that is.) Josh was always quite calm about all these new medical developments while one attack followed another that April. As I remember it, we went to the office for adrenalin shots at least four times or more in ten days.

When our pediatrician decided to run a class for parents of children with asthma, our names were high up on the list of candidates for this series of meetings. Even as he worked on evaluating Josh's medication almost day-by-day, adding, changing, deleting, improving, listening to those lungs and listening again, our worst fears were alleviated by these wonderful classes. After hearing what some of the other parents had been through and were going through, we realized that Josh was not so badly off as we had thought. I can't ever tell you what a relief it was to finally, once and for all, understand that Josh would not die in the ten minute interval between our house and the doctor's office, no matter how bad he sounded.

We learned about all of the different kinds of asthma medicines, how they work, why they are chosen for use. We learned that lung damage before adolescence is rare indeed. We began to face the probability that Josh would remain medicated for years, and that he might not ever "outgrow" it, although no one could predict anything and I still, to this day, hope that he will. We learned how to judge the severity of an attack by looking at the retractions at his neck. We were taught how to use the stethoscope and urged to buy one and were instructed in its use as a diagnostic tool at home. And then came the endless (or so it seemed) months of keeping a record, listening three times a day, writing down in a sort of code a day-by-day description of his condition. Figuring out the inspiration-expiration ratios when he was ill, etc.

I began to feel that I was partly the doctor. There were many consultations (by phone and in the office) during this initial period of treatment--perhaps stretched over a year or more. At last we arrived at an effectve combination of long-acting theophylline, metaproteronol and anti-histamine. During this time, our pediatrician seemed constantly to be attending seminars on this stubborn disease, and trying new ideas. He liberalized his attitude toward the inhaler, and taught us to use it as a preventive tool right along with the other medication. I think that was the final refinement, and it serves us in good stead. Our rule is that Josh may use the inhaler three times a day, but after that the doctor wants to hear about it and, most likely, to see him. This has almost never occurred.

It came as a big surprise to me when, last year, I had to be reminded that it was time to bring Josh in for a checkup. He had been going to the doctor's so often, it never occurred to me that three months might slip by without a visit.

Josh underwent another series of allergy tests, but no strategic information turned up. Several times he underwent theophylline blood-level tests, which revealed that he seemed to metabolize the stuff at an awesome rate. He began taking it in 400 mg. doses twice a day which I thought was enough to kill a horse, but seemed finally to be just right for treating a 70 lb. boy.

This May, when a late spring caught up with Josh and I brought him in wheezing badly, it came as quite a surprise even to the doctor to see by the record that Josh had not been in for an adrenalin shot in over a year.

I attribute a lot of this good track record to intelligent and discriminating use of the inhaler. Josh has learned to carry it with him when he goes fishing (which is any time the sun shines and the temperature is above freezing, all year round), when he plays soccer, and when he travels anywhere at all. The inhaler seems to nip things in the bud. One of the most important things I remember learning from the Parents' Asthma Group is how one attack triggers another, leaving the lungs in a susceptible condition for maybe 48 hours after the symptoms appear to have gone. This placed the prophylactic approach in context for me and helped me to accept it.

I finally rebelled against record keeping after Josh had been quite well for a long time. I put away my stethoscope several years ago (although it is always there if I need it). I have learned to get all the lung information I need by pressing my ear right up to a bare chest. From time to time, I hear that damned wheezing, in a very small way; usually right before the eight o'clock medicine.

The most interesting thing is how Josh is completely in control of his own medication. I have nothing to do with it. The school nurse never calls me any more. Josh leaves me a note when it is time to refill the prescription. He had dropped his three o'clock metaproteronol and allergy pill for several months over the summer. Just yesterday, I saw a big note that he left for himself on the kitchen counter near his pills:

JOSH TAKE YOUR THREE O'CLOCK PILLS

Once in a while there are complications. Just two days ago, he forgot he had taken his evening medicine and took it again. He was up a good part of the night vomiting and enduring stomach pain. Occasionally this theophylline reaction occurs for no obvious reason--he just is temporarily more sensitive I guess. That's my educated guess, of course. For I am, after all, an educated parent. With an educated asthma child. I wouldn't have it any other way.

P.S. Josh is now in the fifth grade, reading on an early sixth-grade level. He repeated a year, and thanks to the superb special ed teachers and resource room attention, in combination with correct medication, he is now, this year, fully back in the classroom with no special aid. He is a happy and highly motivated boy.

RYAN

Living With Fast Asthma

By Dana Parker

Just before Thanksgiving of '81, our son Ryan caught a cold, and developed a really bad cough. Since he was only three we were concerned about him, and gave him a standard dose of kid's aspirin, cough medicine, and sent him to bed. At 3 a.m. he was worse. His eyes were puffy and red, his cough was worse and his breathing was shallow. These symptoms had no special meaning for us. We saw the pediatrician later that morning. He decided Ryan had asthma and began a course of treatment that is etched in my memory in a way that reminds me of how much we learned, how scared we were, and by contrast how differently we handle the problem now. This first time though, Ryan had gotten in deep. After six hours in the treatment room at the doctor's office, where he had received four shots of adrenalin, vomited oral medication five times and received an hour of intravenous theophylline treatment, our limp and exhausted three-year-old son went to the hospital.

He stayed in the hospital for a couple of days, and we shared 24-hour companionship with our son through the ordeal, until he came home. Almost immediately I began learning about this thing asthma. I was being asked to quickly learn as much as I could digest about the problem, starting with making a regular assessment of our son's medical condition, and feeding that back to the doctor. We were told that we had the best tools for noting and reporting small but significant changes in Ryan's condition both in a measurable clinical way, and also in that indeterminable way that parents look at their children. We can tell the quality of how the kid feels by the color in his face, the way he speaks and the "droop" of his eyes. Almost overnight we became experts at assessing his condition by looking at the retraction of the soft fleshy skin, by carefully listening to I/O ratios, by counting respirations, and listening to the wheeze.

We learned from each of the five asthma attacks that Ryan had over the next four months. Our whole family read the book, Teaching Myself About Asthma, and the 20 or so handouts that our doctor demanded that we learn cold. The short course we participated in with other parents of kids with asthma was a big help in tying things together. This education works, for in spite of the subsequent episodes, Ryan has not been back to the hospital.

The way that we have come to treat the problem at our house has developed quite quickly from panic and fear, into a pretty manageable ritual. Certainly after that first trip to the hospital, we were bound and determined to do better next time. The hospital was the last place I wanted to be with Ryan, unless we had no choice. We were told quite to our amazement that kids don't often require hospitalization, and that indeed, Ryan had a real bad episode. He is a kid that gets in trouble quickly, and we had to move just as quickly to help. It is clear that the treatment team consists of the three doctors, my wife and I, Ryan, and our other sons. The clinical assessment of the I/O ratio, retractions, rate of respiration, and wheezing has become something that we do out of habit, sometimes several times a day, often 30 times a day during an attack. We do it because we now know what Ryan looks like before he's going to have an asthma attack. He also knows how he feels when it's coming on, because his brother reads the asthma book to him a lot. Although he's only a couple of months short of four now, he can tell you what happens to his bronchial tubes during an attack, and he gets out his big graduated pitcher for drinks because he knows he needs a lot of liquids to get better. And medication.

You know, Ryan is weird. He battled over taking the Gyrocaps; he threw up over the issue of taking medicine at all for a long time. But he loves to take what we have finally arrived at: liquid theophylline. When medicine is essential to recovery, it gets important to me... to the point of being crazy. He hated the capsules so badly, and refused to take enough into his system voluntarily. One day I set him in the high chair with the sole intention of getting those meds into the kid. He won. We stayed in that kitchen for most of the day, and he would not comply. My panic was due to my memory of what happens when a kid doesn't take medicine... he gets worse and goes to the hospital. Finally, out of desperation, we called the doctor and we changed the meds to liquid... all is fine, and has been since the end of the first attack.

Certainly our view was that we would prefer to have Ryan at home, and not at the hospital, or even over at Amherst Medical if we could help it. What has developed over the last six months is absolutely terrific. Through the work with the pediatric staff and through our shared assessment of our son an interesting working relationship has developed. We have incredible confidence in our three pediatricians, and they have confidence in us. They trust and confirm our judgment, over the phone. We often call and check in during an attack, or when we get concerned, and we confer about issues of how serious the symptoms, medication levels, complications, and ultimately the decision about where he needs to be cared for. As a result, we make fewer trips to the doctor's office, we feel more able to help Ryan directly, and we feel much more confident in trusting ourselves. We take good care of Ryan, and make sound medical judgments with "good supervision." Because we have learned an accurate and common medical language, that supervision can take place over the phone. This has helped us move from feeling helpless and a victim of the illness, to being an active part of the getting better. We also have become more aware of the things that trigger Ryan's asthma. When Ryan has a cold, we start the meds. When it's below 32 degrees out, he wears a mask, and is only out for brief periods of time. On his own, Ryan avoids dusty and "bad air" situations. He doesn't like to have attacks either.

As a family, we have struggled with this thing. I think we are winning. Issues of attention to the other children have come up. Trying to do things like work, stay normal, sleep at night, not argue due to our overtiredness, control the anger which comes from old impressions of asthma which remain... this is hard work. The results however have been gratifying. We are delighted that we can call Amherst Medical, get through to a doctor who knows us well and trusts our judgment. We are surprised at how many trips to the office we have avoided, and how reassuring it is for Ryan to be in his own house, his own bed, hearing the familiar sounds of home.

You also should know that Ryan, in spite of his asthma, and in spite of how quickly he gets in trouble (2-6 hours after the first obvious signs) is a tough, active athletic little kid. He climbs anything with a foothold, runs like the wind, and rarely tires.

I firmly believe that while the problem is scary and quite serious, it is quite understandable. We could have remained victims of the panic, and have the fear that we could not help our son, but we have not. We hope that Ryan's body will begin to grow in a predictable way, that his windpipes will enlarge significantly, and therefore relieve some of the problem. This may happen around the ages of 4-6. If the asthma continues, we know how to help him, and he is getting better at knowing how to help himself.

We don't know everything about asthma, but we know a lot about our son's asthma. We all work hard at it, and the panic is gone from the situation. We feel pretty good about how we handle it, and it makes Ryan feel better when we can show him that confidence.

MATTHEW

By Jeamie Duffy

Since Matthew was one year old I had it in the back of my mind to write something about asthma for parents, even if it were just a list of our experiences and feelings. I see asthma as a family illness and a family affair. It affects the entire family not just the person who has it. The interactions between two parents and between parents and child affect every family. They take on added significance when your child has asthma.

Matthew's story really begins before his birth. My husband and I both have asthma and were prepared for an allergic child. I have outgrown my asthma; my husband however would be called moderately severe to this day. My father, a physician, warned us when we were first married to carefully consider the decision to have children because of our allergic histories. Luckily, we followed our desire to have at least one child.

Because we were prepared, his bedroom was never cluttered with stuffed animals, toys or knickknacks. There were never any animals to remove from our home. His bedroom contained a crib, a dresser and a lamp. To this day it remains the same.

Matthew's first sign of trouble came when he was about five months old. He was lying on the floor, munching on a cracker when all of a sudden I heard that very familiar wheeze. I have to emphasize that we were ready for this. I knew what wheezing sounded like. I knew that he would <u>not</u> stop breathing. I knew he needed to be treated. In this sense, we were lucky. I can imagine the frightening feeling of seeing and hearing your infant have trouble breathing and not knowing exactly what was happening or what to do.

The first episode was mild. Liquid theophylline for a few days was all that he needed. The largest problem was convincing the doctor that he had asthma. He had trouble believing that Matthew's trouble would start so early or that the parents could diagnose the problem themselves. By the time he was a year old, Matt had maybe two more mild episodes and we had moved to Amherst, Mass. By then he was on a maintenance dose of theophylline and was becoming quite allergic. He was underweight and had "the look." He often had allergic shiners, got eczema from certain foods and constantly had a stuffy nose.

My first scare came when he was about eighteen months old. Matthew was playing in our backyard one spring afternoon. I looked out to find him "groping" toward the house. He had come in contact with some grass or bushes and had then rubbed his eyes. His eyes were swollen to the point of distortion and the lower membrane was so swollen that I could not see the eyeball. I was not ready for this! No matter how prepared I was for an allergic child, this was too much--because I didn't know what to do. A single dose of anti-histamine cleared up the problem and we had one more bit of information for future reference.

The interplay of medications is a tricky business. It was not until recently that we realized that certain antibiotics may raise the theophylline level to toxicity. When your child takes four different medications, you become a juggler, trying to give them at different intervals so as not to upset the stomach. More on medicines later.

By age two, Matthew's asthma was getting worse, as was my husband's. That spring was bad! Matthew spent Mother's Day at the hospital with a full-fledged attack and I was beginning to get upset. My husband Joe would go to the emergency room one evening, and a few days later Matthew would follow. I once remarked to my mother that I was hearing stereo wheezing throughout the house.

At this time, I was beginning to let Matthew's asthma become the focal point in my life. This obsession, which I will admit is natural, lasted for about two and a half years. In retrospect, it was not good for anyone. My obsession took the form of over-protection and his illness was constantly on my mind. I was afraid to let him near a child with a cough for fear he'd catch cold. I was afraid to let him near an animal for fear it would trigger his wheezing.

I became compulsive about keeping the house clean. I would dust and vacuum every day to attain the perfect dust-free environment. While this effort can be very important with an allergic child, I went overboard. To this day, I do try to keep a clean house, but the cleaning has gone to every other day and even a third day when necessary. Now I clean because I want to have a dust-free home, not because I'm driven to keep a dust-free home.

I was also beginning to feel very sorry for myself. I would talk about Matthew's problem to anyone who would listen. Each asthma attack was repeated in the last detail to friends, family and even strangers. I needed to talk about his problem to "get it off my chest." Yes, his asthma was bad, but I seemed to make it appear worse as I talked about it to friends. As I look back, I think I wanted sympathy. After an attack, I would be very tired from lots of sleepless nights and wanted someone to take care of me for a while. Trying to be Super Mom is exhausting!

Joe and I never disagreed about Matthew's health. We reacted to it differently. He never went to the extremes that I did. One of the reasons I think this was so is because he worked and I didn't. He could walk away in the morning to an exciting (seemingly so) job and away from Matt's health. I, on the other hand, was surrounded by his illness. He was not in school so I had nothing to divert my attention. Each cough meant another attack--more adrenalin--more nights awake--the circle never stopped.

This was also the time when we began to discuss our family size. We had always said that we wanted two kids. By this time, I was questioning whether we wanted another. Joe was too. I couldn't see having another child with asthma. It was expensive, it was tiring, it was emotionally draining. We decided against another child. Rather, we put off thinking about it for a while. The discussion would come up every six months or so, always with the same results--let's wait.

When Matthew was three, he needed his first dose of steroids. I don't think I will ever forget that day. It was the 4th of July weekend--we were playing "hide and seek" and I could easily find Matthew by listening for his wheeze and cough. After a few shots of adrenalin, it was obvious that he needed something more. He began his first course of prednisone. To me, that meant that he had reached another level of his illness--a more serious level. Prior to this, shots of adrenalin would break an attack. Now we were bringing in the "big guns."

We knew about prednisone and that it could be potentially dangerous. It is a very scary feeling to give your child a drug that could retard growth, eat away at calcium deposits, cause bones to become fragile and easily broken, and yet know that your child has to have it. We would cross our fingers as we gave him the medication, and pray that we were doing the right thing. Sure, the doctor can prescribe the pills and tell you that your child needs it, but it is you who wonders what those side effects will do to your child. Joe and I worried that he might not grow to his expected potential.

Throughout all this, Matthew was growing up to be a happy, normal child. He took his illness in stride. As a matter of fact, he never thought of himself as being ill. He thought all kids took medicine every day. He thought everyone's eyes itched when near animals. He thought everyone needed shots to help them breathe. His dad did all these things--why not everyone?

Joe and I strongly believed that if we raised him as a child with a chronic illness, he would grow up with an emotional illness too. We were straightforward about what restrictions he had (food, animals, etc.) but we spoke of these in the same tone that we warned him about playing with matches. He never saw himself as being different. We always let him determine how much physical activity he could handle. We never stopped him from playing ball, running or other vigorous activities. There were times when I wanted to. There were times when maybe we should have. But we felt that if we interfered, he and his friends would think of him as being different. Then he could always have a crutch when things did not go his way. "I'm wheezy and I can't go to bed," "I have asthma, therefore I need and deserve special attention."

There was one time when I especially wanted to stop him. There was a group of children playing tag in our front yard. One child was "it" while the rest ran around not to get caught. Matthew was having trouble with his asthma and was still playing. But he never moved. He ran in place, or rather moved in place. He never moved from that one spot. None of the children realized what he was doing, but I watched from the front window. Our child refused to be different, our child refused to be sick. Matthew was "one of the kids." I wanted to stop that game and start a quiet one, but I stayed out. It was important for Matthew to learn to make judgments and set the limits.

Joe and I are very proud of the fact that Matthew does not feel sorry for himself or think of himself as being different. It is hard not to buy some special toy when he is sick; it is hard not to wait on him hand and foot when he is having an attack. You want to do special things, yet when a child has a chronic illiness you would always be doing that special thing. Then you're in trouble. I remember when Matthew was three and a half he had an espcially bad attack that lasted days, with numerous trips to the doctor and a lot of shots. This was the time Matthew first asked for a Big Wheel. During the attack, I wanted to go out and buy the Big Wheel and tell him he was so good about the shots and all that we bought him the bike. Instead, we waited for about three weeks and then gave it to him, saying we were proud of him and that he was a good boy. He knew he was getting rewarded for being good, not for being sick.

The regimen of medication was becoming difficult at this time. He was now taking prednisone frequently and this presented a problem. Prednisone only comes in pill form and Matthew did not swallow pills yet. This meant crushing the pill and mixing it with applesauce. A crushed prednisone pill tastes worse than a crushed aspirin (I know because I tried it). Not only did he have to take these during the day, but we had to wake him at night and feed this mixture to him. He would wake up, eat the applesauce, shudder at the taste, and go right back to sleep. There was never any crying or complaining. We were also having to wake him up at night to give his theophylline, so each night meant at least one interruption of sleep.

The other aspect of all the medication was the behavior changes which theophylline caused, i.e., nervousness and jumpiness. Prednisone can cause mood swings (high and low). Matthew gets exuberant on the prednisone and we recognized this right away. Metaproterenol tablets caused his hands to shake. All of this creates a problem with discipline. If Matthew acted up, being fresh or belligerent, we felt at times that it was because of the medication. But we also felt that the behavior had to be stopped. If he got away with this behavior while on medication, he would surely try while off it. It is difficult to punish your child for something he might not have control over--but you know you must.

Other people's reactions to Matthew were quite varied. A few examples can best show this (the good and the bad). When Matthew was about three and a half, we went to the grocery store soon after an attack. However, even though the wheezing had stopped, his cough continued. Matthew's cough is loud and deep. There was one time when he broke a few blood vessels in his face from coughing so hard. While we were shopping, he started to cough. A woman passed me in the aisle, listened to Matthew, and shook her head. We passed her again a few aisles later and Matthew was still coughing. The woman stopped me and asked how I had the nerve to take such a sick child outside. At first I wanted to explain, then I wanted to yell at her that it was none of her business. I did neither. She walked away shaking her head, probably thinking I was an incompetent mother. I left angry!

Another time at the movies, because of Matthew's coughing the people behind us got up and moved. I'm sure they were afraid their child would catch some horrible disease. I didn't blame them, for I probably would have done the same thing. However, it is embarrassing. When Matthew is coughing, people give us looks as if that child belongs in the hospital, not at the Mall. I have even considered getting a T-shirt printed with, "I'm not sick or contagious, it's just my asthma."

But for every embarrassing situation, there are many more just the opposite. Our next door neighbors have a boy just Matthew's age and they became best friends. They have a cat which means that Matthew can never go inside their house to play. Spring and summer are no problem, but winter is hard. After Matthew had to miss Ray's birthday party because of the cat, they gave the cat away. I hope I never forget the feeling I got when Dottie told me why they gave the cat away. She said that Matthew and Ray's friendship was more important and would last longer than the cat. Of course, we never asked them or expected them to do so. They realized on their own how hard it was on Matthew. There also have been many situations when people have given birthday parties at McDonalds, because Matthew couldn't come to a home with pets.

In the spring when Matthew was about four, he had a very bad time. We seemed to be at the doctor's office every day and sometimes twice a day. Luckily, at this time he learned to swallow pills and to use an inhaler, which made medicating easier. His asthma seemed to be getting worse. I was very down. Part of my depression I'm sure came from lack of sleep, but I also saw this illness as an ongoing thing which I could not keep up with. Sure an attack would subside, but sure also was the fact that he would have another soon. I talked about it with my dad who is a pediatrician. He told us that very soon Matthew would outgrow his problem, or at least get much better. Sure enough, he did. From that spring for the next ten months, Matthew had very little trouble. He was still taking daily medication, but each cold now did not trigger an attack. We were thrilled. We were even ready to consider having another child. I was convinced that Matthew was outgrowing his asthma and would soon be fine. We were even talking to the doctor about tapering him off his daily medications.

This interlude did not last. The next spring came along and Matthew was even worse. Again, there were multiple attacks and trips to the doctor. I felt crushed. I had emotionally convinced myself that Matthew was better. Now, besides having to deal with an attack, I had to face the fact that he had not outgrown the problem. It was a double whammy that spring. It took a long time for me to get out of the depression. Probably the best thing I did was to get a part-time job when he started kindergarten.

With a new job, I had more to think about than a clean house, Matthew's cough and juggling medicines. My work in the morning while he was in school gave me an outlet for my energy and a new focus for my thought. At this time, my obsession with Matthew's health began to subside. It was not an immediate thing, but a gradual lessening of my emotional involvement. Over a period of months I began to accept the fact that Matthew had a chronic illness, but not a debilitating one. Yes, he was limited in certain things, but taken as a whole he was able to live a normal life and so should I. Of course, Joe and I were still concerned when he had an attack, but we also knew that he would come out of it and go right back to being an active, happy boy. He still took a lot of medication, but now it was much easier. We had worked out a comfortable schedule for medication. He had to take a theophylline capsule at 4:00 p.m. every day. The neighbors used to say they could set their clocks by the time I got on my bike with pill and water, trying to find Matthew who was playing outside. We no longer had to wake him during the night to give medication: he got a larger dose before bed--therefore we all slept better.

When Matthew was five and a half, he required hospitalization for an attack. He began to cough a little on a Tuesday, three days before we were to go to New Jersey to visit relatives. We heard him cough and waited. By the next day, the cough was getting worse but not bad enough to call the doctor. That night, I turned to Joe and said, "I'll bet he has an attack by Friday, when we're supposed to leave." Sure enough, he did. We went to New Jersey anyway, but had to turn around and come back the next morning. Joe's aunt, a nurse, said she didn't think he was <u>that</u> bad and why were we going home. We knew. Six hours later, he was in the hospital with the worst attack ever. I bring this up to show that parents know what is going on with their kid. You develop a sixth sense about your child and his health. The doctors we take Matthew to believe that parents who know what is happening are the best diagnosticians for their child. Thanks to them, we know how medications work, what their side effects are and how to judge the severity of an attack. We know how to determine if he is getting worse and what action to take. Put simply, we know what to do. I can honestly say that I know when Matthew is getting bad even before the actual signs appear. People (and doctors) ask what it is that tells me this. I cannot put it into words. It's a combination of the way he acts and the way he looks. If we took him to the doctor when I sensed that he was getting bad, probably the doctor would not hear a lot of wheezing or see outward signs. Luckily, our doctors trust us as parents and listen to us. I feel Matthew has been kept healthier because of this.

The hospitalization at age five was probably less traumatic than previous attacks. Sure, it hurt with an IV and lots of blood tests, but I did not get depressed and Matthew did not get upset. Whenever Matthew has to undergo an uncomfortable procedure (i.e., blood test), he never cries or complains. I believe he sensed that this was what he needed to get better. I am not the religious type, but I do believe God gives children with chronic illnesses a little extra something. That something might take the form of patience or acceptance.

Since then, Matthew has been scratch tested for allergies (we were not surprised when he showed up positive) and begun allergy shots. I can't say that we've seen any improvement, but we're still trying. His asthma has not gotten any better, but he is better controlled with medication. Therefore, the attacks are less frequent and more easily controlled.

Matthew is seven now. He had to be hospitalized again recently but for only three days. And how quickly he bounces back! The afternoon of his discharge, he was out riding his bike.

Sure, Joe and I still have our moments of being down, and there are times when I want to start feeling very sorry for myself and Matthew; but when those feelings begin I look at our family as a whole and have to be happy. As I finish this story, Matthew is out in the front yard with ten neighbors playing baseball. He is a happy child—full of fun and energy. He can do all those "normal" things. If he starts to wheeze while playing, he just calls 'time out', comes in to use his inhaler, and runs back out again.

NATHAN

By Marilyn Sansouci

Our fourth son Nathan was born in April 1981. He weighed 8 lbs., 10 oz. and was a very handsome little fellow. We were very pleased with him. He was healthy and fine until one day in November when he caught a cold. We treated it with aspirin and decongestant. This didn't seem to help him at all. By the third day he became worse. He began to cough quite frequently and he was breathing rapidly. By the time evening came, our baby was struggling to breathe. We immediately called an ambulance which took us to the hospital. He was put in an oxygen tent for several days. After taking chest x-rays, the doctor said that our son had pneumonia. He gave him an antibiotic and after a week's stay in the hospital, Nathan was sent home. He did fine for three weeks but when he caught another cold, it turned into a nightmare.

Late one night I had awakened out of a sound sleep with a feeling that I should look in on the baby. I check on all the boys every night (a mother's routine) before I go to bed, but this time it was different. When I went into Nathan's room I heard him wheezing and coughing and gasping for air. I ran and woke my husband. We rushed our baby to the hospital and on the way total fear gripped me. I feared that this time we were going to lose our son. By the time we got to the hospital, Nathan's lips began to turn blue from lack of oxygen. He again was put into an oxygen tent, and all we could do was pray to God that our baby would be all right. I believe it was a miracle, an answer to prayer, that Nathan did survive. They took more chest x-rays and did a test for cystic fibrosis which was negative and we were very thankful for that.

I remember feeling distressed and questioning how long this would continue to go on before we would find out what was causing our little boy to get so sick so often. When I was to bring Nathan home from the hospital approximately one week later, I called his doctor to ask if he had made a diagnosis yet. He told me there was still no diagnosis and encouraged me just to be happy he was better. Well, by this time I had had my fill of finding out nothing concerning my baby. Certainly we were happy that he was better, but for how long? We knew something was terribly wrong but we just didn't know what. We decided it was time to change doctors. At this time we were referred to another pediatrician by a friend. The first time we visited this new doctor and I told him of Nathan's trauma, he diagnosed him as having asthma and began treatment with theophylline three times a day. In spite of this treatment, Nathan was still hospitalized two more times before his first birthday.

In March of 1982 we joined a health maintenance organization. The next time Nathan had an asthma attack, he was examined by our new family doctor, who then phoned for a pediatric consultation. After he got off the phone he ordered three shots for Nathan. I believe the shots were adrenalin twice, followed by Sus-Phrine. Nathan responded and was able to go home within an hour. He continued treatment with theophylline capsules and prednisone three times a day for a short period of time. This was the first time that he had an attack and was not admitted. We were so thrilled to be able to take our baby home the same night. It was beautiful not to have to go home to an empty crib. This was also the beginning of learning about our son's asthma.

Nathan was fine for about a month and then he had another attack. This time the pediatrician increased the theophylline dose but Nathan couldn't tolerate the full amount. He got hyperactive and wouldn't sleep at night. He did calm down after it was reduced. The consulting pediatrician prescribed metaproterenol followed by cromolyn, both delivered by powered nebulizer three times a day. This amounts to a regular program of treatment and prevention at the same time.

Not long ago my family doctor recommended that my husband and I attend the Parents' Asthma Group that was held in Amherst. We attended two two-hour sessions and are very glad we did. We learned a lot about asthma and how to detect attacks early and how to monitor these attacks. We also learned about various medicines used to treat asthma, their good effects and also the undesirable effects. It was good to share experiences with other parents: what they were going through, how they were dealing with it, what their feelings were about asthma and how it affected them. It helps to know that we are not the only parents going through these problems. It is important to hear how others deal with this important issue.

In the beginning of Nathan's sickness, we feared for his life. At the Parents' Asthma Group we learned that it was rare for a child to die of asthma. Only one of every 25,000 children with asthma die of it each year. If parents have adequate knowledge and see that their children get proper treatment, this tiny number will become smaller still.

Nathan is now three years old and doing much better. In the two years he has been on this new treatment plan, he hasn't been admitted to the hospital once. He takes theophylline capsules twice a day except when he begins a cold, then I'll add another capsule at night. He takes metaproterenol and cromolyn by nebulizer three times a day. Since we've learned more about how to deal with Nathan's condition and he's on this medication, he has gone as long as three months without an attack. Before he was having them at least once a month. What an improvement!

CHAPTER TWO

THE BASICS

You need some basic information before you can take care of your child's asthma. This chapter provides the basics and some tools to judge what is going on in an asthma attack. Once you can judge the severity of an attack and understand the importance of keeping an asthma record, you have a foundation on which you can build.

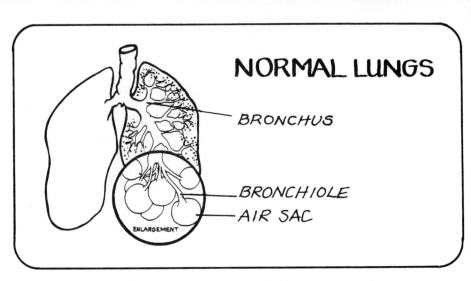

NORMAL LUNGS

— BRONCHUS

— BRONCHIOLE
— AIR SAC

ENLARGEMENT

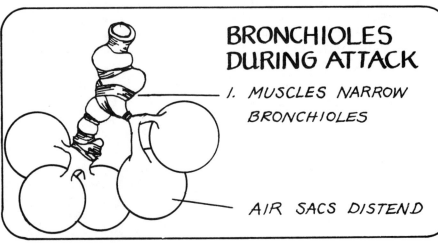

BRONCHIOLES
DURING ATTACK

1. MUSCLES NARROW
BRONCHIOLES

AIR SACS DISTEND

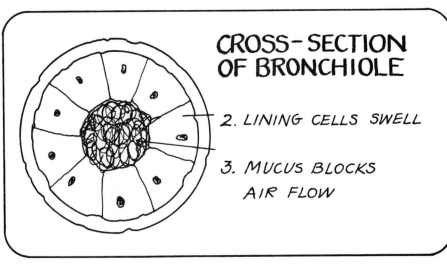

CROSS-SECTION
OF BRONCHIOLE

2. LINING CELLS SWELL

3. MUCUS BLOCKS
AIR FLOW

WHAT IS ASTHMA?

Asthma is a disease in which the windpipes over-react. It is known to some as bronchitis, wheezy bronchitis, bronchial asthma and asthmatic bronchitis. Doctors call it reversible obstructive airway disease. This indicates that the windpipes become temporarily narrowed or blocked but can recover.

How do the windpipes get narrowed or blocked?

The windpipes become blocked three different ways in an asthma attack. First, the muscles encircling the windpipes tighten and thus narrow the air passage. Second, the cells lining the windpipe swell and narrow it still further. Third, these same cells secrete mucus which can plug the remaining opening in the windpipe. Except for the muscle tightening, it is much like what happens in your nose with a cold.

What is an asthma attack?

An asthma attack is any episode of asthma that involves worsening of breathing that interrupts on-going activities or requires some procedure, such as resting or taking medicine, before one can resume normal and comfortable breathing.

What triggers an asthma attack?

Narrowing of the windpipes in a person with over-reactive airways can be set off by any number of triggers.

What are some of the triggers?

Viral respiratory infections, such as colds, sinusitis and bronchitis, are the most common triggers of asthma. Exercise, especially in cold weather, often sets off asthma. A change in the weather may lead to an attack. Pollutants, such as cigarette smoke, perfumes, dust and chemicals, also trigger asthma. Allergens (any substances which are capable of producing allergic responses or symptoms, for example, dust, pollens, molds, animal dander) are significant triggers in about 10% of our patients. Emotions are rarely a factor in triggering an attack unless they lead to an outburst of yelling, crying, screaming or laughing. These activities themselves can provoke an attack.

Does every attack need treatment?

In general, yes. The severity of an attack is not predictable at the outset. Medications are less effective as the attack progresses. Early, aggressive treatment is the mainstay of effective management.

JUDGING THE SEVERITY OF YOUR CHILD'S ASTHMA ATTACK

Emlen Jones, M.D.

It is usually obvious when a child is having an asthma attack, but sometimes difficult to tell how serious a particular attack is. Older children will tell you how they feel and can compare it with previous occurrences. Younger children may just "not act themselves" and have breathing difficulties.

When a child with asthma is evaluated by a physician, certain characteristics of his/her breathing are looked at carefully. In the table below, we list three types of observations that are valuable in judging the severity of an asthma attack. Using these you can grade attacks as mild, moderate, or severe.

Severity of Asthma Attack	I:O Ratio	Wheezing	Retractions
Mild	Near normal 1.5:1	Mild expiratory	None
Moderate	Approximately 1:1	Full Expiratory	Mild
Severe	Less than 1:1	Inspiratory & marked expiratory	Marked

I:O Ratio: This is the best way to tell how your child is doing. It is a measure of how long breathing in lasts as compared to breathing out. Breathe in and out with your child to get the feel of it. In the normal breathing pattern, breathing in lasts 50% longer than breathing out (1.5:1). When an asthma attack occurs it takes longer to breathe out (O). In a mild attack, the difference is hardly noticeable. In a moderate attack, in and out become about equal (I:O equals 1:1). In a severe attack, breathing out takes longer than breathing in.

Wheezing: This is the high-pitched, whistling sound that occurs when air flows through narrowed bronchial tubes. At the start of an attack the wheezing only occurs when the child is breathing out (expiration). In mild cases, the wheezing occurs at the end of the breathing-out phase. As the attack gets worse, wheezing lasts through all of expiration, and finally occurs when the child is breathing in. Wheezing does not occur in a bronchial tube which is totally blocked. The absence of wheezing in a child who has severe retractions and a reversed I:O ratio (1:2) is a sign of very serious trouble. When this patient improves (reopens some windpipes) wheezing will reappear.

Retractions are the sucking in of the soft tissues in the chest which occurs when there is difficulty breathing. These are first obvious below the rib cage and in the soft part of the neck above the breast bone, as well as in the soft tissue over the collarbone. In more severe cases, the tissue between the ribs may be sucked in. These changes are the measure of the difficulty of breathing and a good guide to the severity of an attack.

Mild asthma attacks should always be treated, but in many families can be handled at home alone or with telephone consultation. Persistence of even mild symptoms for several days should prompt a visit to the physician.

Moderate and severe attacks: if they do not respond to the usual treatments at home within two hours, this should always prompt a telephone call, and usually an office visit without delay.

COMMENT

Once a parent can judge the severity of an attack s/he can get phone advice on the management of an attack from the physician. For example, when Ryan had an attack late one night, his parents started treatment according to a pre-set plan. His dad called me at 9 a.m. to say that Ryan had improved and now his I:O ratio was 1:1.5, he was wheezing in and out, his respirations were 46. I advised him to come in for nebulizer treatment in three hours if he did not improve further. At noon Dad called saying Ryan's I:O ratio was 1:1, he was wheezing less and his respiratory rate was 42. He felt Ryan was definitely better and continued to treat him at home.

Harriet Cohen called one afternoon to say that Josh had started a cold three days ago, then developed a cough and today his I:O was 1:1 and he had a slight expiratory wheeze. He was taking full doses of theophylline and using a metaproterenol inhaler four times a day. She thought he should take a three-day burst of prednisone and wanted to check with me before starting it. Based on her information I agreed that this was the next step.

Eighteen-month Dwayne came to the office one Saturday evening with his first episode of asthma. He was breathing sixty times a minute, had an I:O ratio of 1:1, mild to moderate retractions and was wheezing so loudly I could hear it across the room. As I examined and treated him I reviewed these findings with his parents. Fifteen minutes later he was breathing forty times a minute, his I:O was 1:1, retractions had lessened and the wheeze could only be heard with a stethoscope. Since his attack was moderately severe I asked his parents whether they preferred to observe and treat Dwayne at home or to admit him to the hospital. They felt they could manage at home. When I called them two hours later, Dad reported respirations 48, I:O 1:1, no retraction and slight wheeze. He felt confident that Dwayne's condition was stable. I knew I could count on him to assess the situation until we met the next morning.

A daily record of symptoms, medications and comments has helped me to improve the status of many children with asthma. On entering a new practice five years ago, I found that almost none of the children with asthma were receiving optimal treatment. Their parents usually did not know that certain triggers could provoke an asthmatic attack; also they did not understand the relationship between the dose of a drug and its effect. I spent the greater part of each office visit trying to determine the effects of various triggers and medications on the symptoms of the child with asthma. The parent's recollection was neither complete or precise.

To improve recall, I devised a record for the parent or older child to keep on a daily basis. Now data are collected in advance and we spend the office visit analyzing what happened rather than trying to remember the facts. I can often make informed suggestions for adjusting medications based on the asthma record.

Wheezing, cough, interference with activities and sleep are rated on a daily basis. Medication dose is also listed daily. This record has enabled parents to:

Recall accurately the events which occurred since the last visit by providing a structured format.

Communicate clearly and succinctly on the phone.

Learn when to start medication.

Learn when to reduce medication.

Compare the effects of various dosages and combinations of medications.

Improve treatment since it serves as a reminder to the parent to give medication as directed.

Identify triggers which regularly provoke an attack.

Reduce the duration of the visit and thus the cost of a visit.

Gain an understanding of the pattern of their child's attack.

Become responsible for treatment. The parent is in charge of seeing that the child takes enough medication to be normally active without symptoms. Recording the day's symptoms and level of activities helps parents tune in to their child's condition.

Record and analyze peak flow data.

ASTHMA RECORD - Please bring at each visit

Comment: Many things can trigger an asthma attack including colds or infections, exercise, irritants and allergens. Note any trigger which seems to affect your child the day it occurs. Can you detect any early warning signs which come on before wheezing? Most common are: cough, sneezing, scratchy throat, grumpy.

DATE	WHEEZE	COUGH	ACTIVITY	NIGHT	THEOPHYLLINE	INHALER METAPROTERNOL	PREDNISONE			COMMENTS

-42-

	0	1	2	3
WHEEZE	NONE	Some	Medium	Severe
COUGH	NONE	Occasional	Frequent	
ACTIVITY	NORMAL	Can run short distance	Can walk only	missed school or stayed indoors
NIGHT	FINE	Slept well slightly wheezy	Awake 2-3 times with wheeze	bad night awake most of the time

This 14-year-old girl came to the office because of frequent cough for six days. She had no history of asthma. On exam she coughed every 15 seconds and could not take a deep breath without coughing. Mean peak flow (see p. 148) for her height was 480 liters per minute. Hers was 320. After three whiffs of metaproterenol, spaced two minutes apart, she felt better and her peak flow increased from 320 to 380.

I made a diagnosis of asthma and started her on a metaproterenol inhaler and theophylline 200 mg every 12 hours. After three days she increased the theophylline to 300 mg every 12 hours. When I saw her a week later she coughed only once during a fifteen minute visit. She was cheerful, her lungs were clear as before and her peak flow was 460.

Date	WHEEZE	COUGH	ACTIVITY	NIGHT	THEOPHYLLINE	INHALER		COMMENTS
11/3	0	2	3	3	200 200	✓✓ ✓✓		FEEL like drank coffee - couldn't sleep
11/4	0	1	3	2	200 200	✓✓ ✓✓		caughed more after 2 p.m.
11/5	0	1	3	1	200 200	✓✓ ✓✓		felt pretty good only slight cough
11/6	0	1	1	0	300 300	✓✓ ✓✓		worked outside coughed more.
11/7	0	1	1	0	300 300	✓✓ ✓✓		very tired afternoon
11/8	0	1	1	0	300 300	✓✓ ✓✓		felt good - a little trouble in gym
11/9	0	1	0	0	300 300	✓✓ ✓✓		

Her asthma record demonstrates:
- side effect of wakefulness due to theophylline. This was a problem only on the first day
- clear improvement after dose of theophylline was increased on fourth day
- exercise during an attack may increase symptoms

Without a written record, it would be impossible to remember the changes in cough, activity and sleeping in this detail. This teenager learned about her medication and her asthma by producing and analyzing the Asthma Record.

A six-year-old boy with a long history of asthma came to the office because of a cold for one week and a cough for several days. Exam showed some wheezing and a reduced peak flow rate. I prescribed long-acting theophylline every 12 hours, metaproterenol syrup every six hours and a metaproterenol inhaler. His mother phoned with a progress report three days later stating that he had no wheeze or cough and that his activity and sleeping were now normal. She had used the inhaler for only one day and discontinued metaproterenol by mouth after two days. We decided to give only one dose of theophylline the next day and then stop. Mike remained assymptomatic and off all asthma medication.

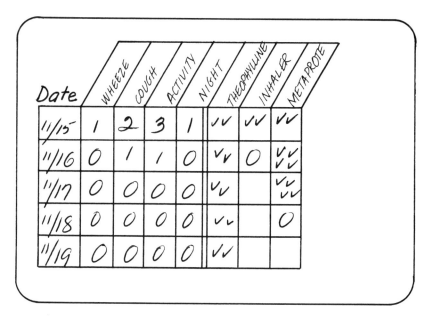

Date	WHEEZE	COUGH	ACTIVITY	NIGHT	THEOPHYLLINE	INHALER	METAPROTE
11/15	1	2	3	1	✓✓	✓✓	✓✓
11/16	0	1	1	0	✓✓	0	✓✓ ✓✓
11/17	0	0	0	0	✓✓		✓✓ ✓✓
11/18	0	0	0	0	✓✓		0
11/19	0	0	0	0	✓✓		

This asthma record helped his mom:

- to recall events accurately
- to learn when to reduce medication
- to communicate clearly and succinctly on the phone
- to learn from the experience of this attack

The most common triggers (substances or events) which provoke asthma attacks are exercise, viral infections, pollutants, cold air, allergens and change in weather.

Hyper-reactivity (sensitivity) of the airways varies greatly from person to person. Some children get an asthma attack only with exercise and not from contact with any of the other usual triggers. A very reactive child may have an attack with each of the triggers mentioned above. The attack may be worsened by the presence of several triggers at the same time. Some children have an attack only when two triggers occur simultaneously, such as exercise or exposure to smoke during a viral infection.

In the graph below you can see that Bob has mildly reactive airways. Exercise alone with not trigger an attack, but exercise in cold air will. Amy is very sensitive to a number of triggers and gets an attack with a viral infection, exposure to a pollutant or to a cat.

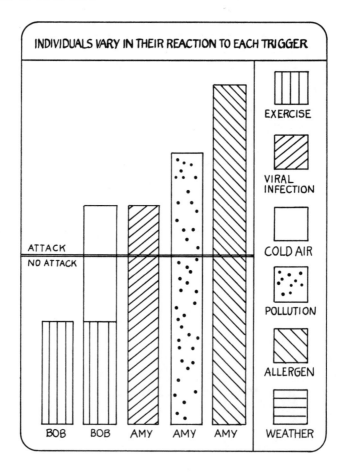

Environmental factors are frequently important triggers in asthma. The vigor of environment controls should match the severity of asthma. Mild asthma may just mean that smoking should not be allowed in the house. Start by making small changes. If you get the desired result, no further changes are necessary. If not, consider taking additional steps to control the environment.

Irritants or pollutants affect everyone's ability to breathe, but patients with asthma often have a more severe reaction to them. The reaction to irritants is added to the reaction that may already exist to an upper respiratory infection, such as a cold or stuffy nose. Some common irritants are dust, mold, deodorants, paint and cigarette smoke.

House dust: These invisible particles come from the breakup of rugs, mattresses, stuffed toys and pets. They float in the air and fall all around. The bedroom is the most important room in the house. In order to properly prepare it and to have a minimum amount of house dust, the following are recommended:
- All sources of dust and dust collectors, including rugs and carpets, should be removed.
- Close all vents, including heating vents, unless air filtration is adequate. If your filtration is good a cheese cloth placed over a vent will stay clean.
- Clean room from top to bottom with a damp mop or cloth once a week. Do not sweep or dry mop since this stirs up dust.

Mold: This is a common irritant. It grows best in damp places and accumulates where there is poor ventilation. We recommend that you:
- keep a light burning in damp closets to prevent mold growth
- avoid raking leaves and harvesting or handling grain or hay.

Temperature: Some patients with winter symptoms do best in cool, moist environments. Bedroom temperature should be 55-60° and the house should be 60-65°.

Effects of strong odors and fumes: Any which you name may cause symptoms. Stay away from hair sprays, perfumes, paints, scented soaps. Sometimes cooking odors cause an asthma attack.

Humidity: The ideal level is 25-40%. This allows enough moisture for the bronchioles to perform their self-cleaning activities. Dry air interferes with this cleaning. Wet air may act as an irritant.

ALLERGY AND ALLERGY SHOTS
Emlen Jones, M.D.

Allergy is an acquired hypersensitivity to a substance (allergen) that does not normally cause a reaction. Symptoms are caused by an antibody reaction which takes place on exposure to the allergen. Frequently this reaction can be confirmed by a positive skin test to the offending substance. Important common allergens include pollens from trees, grasses or weeds, animal danders, dusts and molds.

Asthma is not an allergy. However, allergy does play a significant role in a small percentage (5-10%) of children with asthma. Children whose asthma attacks are consistently related to exposure to some specific substance (for example, dogs, grasses, hay or dust) are likely to have an allergic trigger. Also children who have hay fever (allergic rhinitis), eczema (atopic dermatitis) or other allergic symptoms are also more likely to have allergy involved with their asthma.

Why should we find out if an allergy provokes some of the child's asthma symptoms? Mainly, to advise him to avoid the allergen if it is avoidable. This same philosophy applies to any other trigger of asthma. Also, some children and adolescents may benefit from allergy shots (immunotherapy).

Several studies have confirmed the efficacy of allergy shots in appropriately selected patients. Johnstone, 1968, had followed 210 children for up to 14 years. All had allergy documented by testing. One group got salt water shots, the other group received standard allergy shots. By age 16 years, 22% of the salt water treated children and 72% of the allergy treated children were free of asthma symptoms. A study by Warner in 1978 looked at 85 children who were receiving aggressive drug treatment and who had documented allergy to mite (an imprortant allergen in house dust). Children who had received allergy shots showed a marked decrease of medication use even after a single year of treatment.

Which children with asthma should be investigated for the presence of allergy? I would suggest the following:
- any child with severe asthma, even in the absence of an allergic history. If specific substances are identified which might be factors in asthma, these could be avoided.
- any child with a history that suggests reaction to specific allergens.
- any child with other allergic symptoms, for example, hayfever or eczema.
- certain children with a strong family history of asthma.

How is allergy investigated? A detailed history which includes family and environmental details is taken. This is followed by a careful physical exam to look for any signs of allergy. Laboratory studies usually include a blood count and measurement of IgE, which is an antibody associated with allergy. Various other tests are done in specific circumstances. Finally, skin tests are performed. Small amounts of suspected allergens are either scratched on or injected into the skin and the local reaction is observed.

Not long ago allergy shots were overused in the treatment of asthma. The advent of more effective drug treatment has limited this abuse. We recommend allergy shots (immunotherapy) for children who show significant symptoms to allergens which cannot be avoided. If shots are instituted, they should be continued for a minimum of 2-3 years before deciding whether or not they are helpful. Shots are not given for an allergen which can be avoided, for example, a pet. The shots do not replace standard treatments but are given in addition to these.

EMOTIONS*

Asthma is caused by a complex set of physiological reactions which are not yet completely understood. However, we can say for sure that asthma is not due to a defective mother-child relationship or to any other psychological problem as has been suggested in the past. What role, then, do the emotions play in asthma?

Though emotional factors do not cause asthma they can affect the person with asthma in several ways:

-- The expression of emotions by laughing, crying, or yelling can stimulate the vagus nerve. This causes the muscles around the bronchioles to tighten and starts an attack.

-- Anxiety during an attack may produce hyperventilation which can worsen the attack.

-- Anxiety can cause one person with asthma to assign greater importance to a symptom than would another.

-- The ability to relax may shorten an attack.

-- Patients with chronic asthma sometimes become angry and frustrated and rebel against taking their medications, thus worsening their situation.

-- Some children find that they get special attention when they have an asthma attack. If the benefits outweigh the unpleasantness of an attack, these children may consciously or unconsciously choose to trigger one. Only two of our four hundred patients with asthma seem to have consciously decided that the attention is worth the attack.

What is the effect of asthma on the child's emotions? Children with asthma have been described as depressed, lacking in confidence, or as denying and overcompensating for their illness. I believe that children with asthma have as many different personality types as children without asthma. If a child's asthma is well controlled, as it should be for 99% of children, asthma should play little or no role in his/her psychic functioning.

We find that children who develop asthma in our practice have little difficulty adjusting to it. However, if asthma is not well controlled, the effects on a child's personality may be serious indeed. The same is true for children with other chronic diseases such as diabetes or seizure disorders if they are not well controlled. Some children enter our practice after having

---

*For further discussion see Feelings, p.97

been subjected to years of poorly controlled asthma, punctuated by hospital admissions and numerous trips to the emergency room. These children do fit some of the descriptions of "the asthmatic child." Often they and their parents appear as dependent, helpless individuals who are terrified of the next attack. They have little or no understanding of asthma as a process or what they can and should do about it. Over a period of a year's education and support, most of these children and their parents will learn how to manage their attacks and in the process will become confident controllers of their situation.

In summary:

The disease asthma is not caused by emotional problems.
Emotional events may trigger or worsen an individual asthma attack.
The ability to relax may lessen an attack.
The child whose parents gain a good understanding of asthma and the ability to manage it will only rarely show psychological problems due to the disease.

EXERCISE-INDUCED ASTHMA

Exercise is the most common trigger of asthma. Many people who never wheeze during their usual activities will start to wheeze if they take part in sustained physical activity. Researchers now believe that exercise triggers asthma by lowering the temperature of the windpipes as air exchange increases.

Many children do not know that the tight feeling in their chest can be prevented. Often times a teen with asthma triggered by exercise will restrict his physical activity almost automatically. His parents frequently are not aware that he is limiting himself. They are surprised in the office when their son tells me he doesn't play soccer because he gets a tight chest or starts wheezing after a few minutes of play. Limitation is okay if it is necessary. However, in almost every instance one could prevent the discomfort by proper pre-treatment.

Baseball, football and gymnastics demand less sustained exertion than hockey, soccer, cross country and basketball and are less likely to trigger an attack. Our patients compete in all of these sports. Three of eight players on the first place basketball team in an Amherst league used an inhaler before the game. A mother caught me between periods at a basketball game. She wanted me to know that since her son started using an inhaler before games, he could play a full game. Last year he had to quit at half-time.

The symptoms of exercise-induced asthma usually disappear after two hours if lung function was normal before the exercise. Therefore treatment is much briefer than for an attack of asthma provoked by a viral respiratory infection.

To prevent exercise-induced asthma:
- warm the air by breathing through your nose (a natural air conditioner and warmer)
- create a reservoir of warm air by wearing a painter's or surgeon's mask covered by a scarf when out in cold weather
- use a beta-adrenergic drug or cromolyn by inhaler five minutes before exercise
- use theophylline liquid thirty to sixty minutes before exertion or theophylline tablet an hour before exercise.

COUGHING ASTHMA

Michael Posner, M.D.

Parents usually think of asthma as an illness characterized by labored breathing and wheezing which comes on suddenly as an "attack." In a mild variant form, asthma may come on gradually, may cause no shortness of breath and may cause only a cough which lasts for more than two weeks.

Physicians who study asthma have found that some children have a cough of long duration but with entirely normal physical examinations. Their lung function also is normal. Some of these children will show mild worsening of lung function when they exercise. They may completely lose their coughs when they are placed on standard asthma medication, but begin to cough again after medicine is stopped.

Other children with coughing asthma have chest congestion and sometimes mild wheezing. These children may have reduced lung function. This can be measured in the office and improves with asthma medication.

Both groups of children may develop other symptoms of asthma over time. Other factors considered when diagnosing these mild variants are:
- family history of allergic respiratory conditions
- bronchiolitis in infancy
- shortness of breath with exercise
- past episodes of bronchitis or mild pneumonia
- tendency to prolonged chest colds, especially in spring or fall

There are many children in our practice who have coughs lasting more than two weeks. Some of them may have a mild variant of asthma. If their peak expiratory flow rate (see p. 148) increases 20% or more after inhalation of a beta-adrenergic drug the diagnosis of asthma is clear. For the other children we may suggest a trial of asthma medication. If they improve, they have "coughing asthma" and should take asthma medicine to reduce their cough. Half of these children develop other signs of asthma in a few years. The rest continue to have cough as their only symptom.

NATURAL COURSE OF ASTHMA IN CHILDREN
Emlen Jones, M.D.

Each person has his/her own pattern of asthma both for individual attacks and over a span of years. It is impossible to predict the long term course of asthma symptoms in an individual with accuracy. Some general statements can be made based on research here and abroad. However these studies varied greatly in their definition of asthma and its severity in their subjects.

In the British National Child Development study, researchers checked the records of all children born in England, Scotland and Wales in one week during March 1958. Almost 12,000 children were studied for years. By age seven, three out of every hundred had asthma. Between ages seven and 11 only four new children per thousand developed asthma. Fifty percent of the children whose asthma started before age seven were not wheezing by age eleven. In the United States a study looked at 700 children whose asthma started before age 13. Twenty years later 62 percent of the children without allergies had no symptoms while only 25 percent of the children with allergies lost their symptoms completely. The participants in these studies did not have the benefit of present day treatment. Whether such therapy affects long-term outcome is unknown.

Many children improve between four to six years of age. This is due to a large increase in the size of bronchioles which occurs at this time. However, relapse can occur in adulthood even after long symptom-free periods.

What about severe problems? Death from an acute attack is extremely rare. Improved medications should make even hospitalization unusual. However a child with severe asthma may be hospitalized several times. Severe asthma **does not** usually cause chronic lung disease. Lung damage can occur with cigarette smoking or in high air pollution areas.

Asthma is a common problem. For many children it is chronic and continues into adulthood. When treatment is applied properly the child can lead a normal, productive, well adjusted life. The child with moderate asthma should be able to take part in all social activities and sports unless in the middle of an attack.

Chapter Three
MEDICATIONS

It's easy to treat some problems. For strep throat you just take penicillin three (or four) times a day for ten days. No decisions about how much, how long or whether to use other drugs. And side effects from penicillin are uncommon.

Asthma medications are different. Their dosage has to be adjusted based on symptoms. It can be hard to know when to start and when to stop. Three of the four drug groups cause troublesome side effects.

This chapter outlines when medications should be used, how they affect the windpipes, what trouble they cause and the time factors which apply to each drug. It also includes detailed instructions for using the inhaler since the instructions which come with the inhaler are neither complete nor accurate. "Michelle and the Bubble" describes an inhalation reservoir that is useful for young children. You should ask your doctor to fill out "General Instructions for Treating an Asthma Attack."

You are ready to handle an asthma attack at home if your answers to all the questions in the Asthma Quiz are correct.

The indications and dosages of all drugs in this book have been recommended in the medical literature and conform to the practices of the general medical community. The medications described do not necessarily have specific approval by the Food and Drug Administration for use in the ages and dosages and indications for which they are recommended. The package insert for each drug should be consulted for use and dosage as approved by the FDA. Because standards for usage change, it is advisable to keep abreast of revised recommendations. Consult your physician before making any change in medication.

The four groups of commonly used asthma medications are presented in this section.
- Theophylline type drugs
- Beta-adrenergic, also known as beta-agonist, adrenergic or adrenalin type drugs
- Corticosteroids
- Cromolyn sodium

The time factors section for each drug gives average times. They can vary greatly from one person to another.

As a parent, you have the right and responsibility to know what medicines are being prescribed for your child. In order to be properly informed, you need clear written instructions about any medication your child takes. A list of questions follows. You should be able to answer all of them before you leave the doctor's office.

Questions to Ask About Medications

- What is this drug, and what is it supposed to do?
- Exactly when, and for how long, should I take it?
- What are the possible side effects?
- How long does it take for the medicine to start to work?
- What should I do if it doesn't seem to be working?
- Are there any medicines or foods that I should not use while taking this drug?
- Should this drug be taken before, during or after meals?
- Is there a less expensive form of this drug that I could take?

It is important to take asthma medicine exactly as it is prescribed to have it work correctly. If a medicine is prescribed for every 6 hours, it means every 6 hours, even if that falls in the middle of the night. If that dose is not taken regularly, be sure to let your physician know. He or she may be able to prescribe a longer acting form of the drug.

Brand Names: Many, including Accubron, Ellixophyllin, Slophyllin, Somophyllin, Theodur.

Indications
-- treat asthma attack
-- prevent exercise-induced asthma
-- prevent asthma attack

Desired Effect - Relaxes smooth muscle around the bronchial tubes and so allows them to open more.

Side Effects - Most common side effects are nervousness, overactivity, upset stomach, nausea, vomiting, loss of appetite and headache. These effects often decrease after a few days on the medicine. Theophylline can be irritating to the stomach and should usually be taken with a light snack.

There are many preparations of this drug. Some commonly used ones are:

Form	mg/ml	Comments	Duration
Liquid			
Elixophyllin	5	--	6 Hours
Accubron	10	--	6 Hours
Slophyllin	5	no alcohol	6 Hours
Somophyllin	18	no alcohol	6 Hours
Tablets			
Slophyllin	100,200	scored	6 Hours
Sustained Release			
Slophyllin Gyrocaps	60,125,250	capsule	8 hours
Theodur Tablets	100, 200, 300	scored	12 hours
Theodur Sprinkles	50, 75, 125, 200	capsule	12 hours
Somophyllin CRT	50, 100, 250	capsule	12 hours

We try to use the long-acting preparations for all our patients. Even infants can use capsules. The capsules can be opened and the granules of powder poured into applesauce or a spoon of Redi Whip. A sandwich made of a soda cracker, peanut butter and jelly will disguise the taste. Theodur tablets work well in many children age eight and over. They must be swallowed, not chewed. At the beginning of an attack, plain and sustained release theophylline can be taken together to reach an effective level more quickly for the rare child who needs rapid effect.

Time Factors

Liquid preparations reach an effective level in the blood in thirty minutes. They must be taken every six hours to maintain this level.

Plain theophylline tablets produce an effective blood level in about one hour.

Slophyllin capsules usually produce an effective level after two doses (10 hours) and must be taken every eight hours.

Theodur tablets and sprinkles are sustained release preparations which produce an effective blood level after two doses (13 hours). They must be taken every twelve hours.

Dosage

Doses are individualized but a usual starting dose is 16/mg/kg per day with a maximum of 400 mg per day. The dose is increased by 25% every three days until the desired effect is reached. Once an effective dose is established it can be started immediately for subsequent attacks. Younger children need more theophylline to achieve the desired effect as outlined below:

Under 9 years:	24 mg/kg/day	11 mg/lb/day
9 to 12 years:	20 mg/kg/day	9 mg/lb/day
13 to 16 years	18 mg/kg/day	8 mg/lb/day
17 and over	13 mg/kg/day	6 mg/lb/day

The dose calculations should be based on ideal body weight. This means that an obese child will usually need less medication than a thin child of the same weight.

Some children eliminate this medicine from the body faster than average and will need more of the drug. Viral illnesses and some drugs (for example, erythromycin) slow elimination of theophylline from the body and lower the amount needed. Smoking increases the amount needed.

Sometimes children do not absorb the long-acting theophylline preparations well. When control of asthma is unsatisfactory we measure the amount of theophylline in the blood and then adjust the medication as necessary. A safe effective blood level is between 10 and 20 micrograms per milliliter. If side effects are a problem in this range we consider using another drug.

SWALLOWING PILLS

Some people take the pills and they just slide
But others can't and go and hide
Some think it's torture, and some think it's fun
I think it's better when you're all done

If only I could swallow those pills right down
I would be so happy, just like a clown
I know it's hard, but just try
Don't worry, I even cried

When you're done
You'll see the sun.
Bear with me and try again,
Soon it will work out and that's my plan

--Reneé Cyran

BETA-ADRENERGIC DRUGS BY MOUTH

Metaproterenol
Brand names: Alupent, Metaprel

Indications:
- a child has unacceptable side effects from theophylline and does not have a powered nebulizer at home (about 20% of our patients under three years of age fall into this category).

Desired effect: relaxes smooth muscle around the bronchial tubes and so allows the tubes to open more.

Side effects: usually mild, shakiness, rapid heart beat, pounding in chest, nervousness, nausea, vomiting, headache, pallor.

Form:
- liquid (10 mg/5cc)
- tablet (10 and 20 mg, scored)

Time factors: liquid or tablet takes 30 minutes to work and effect lasts from four to six hours.

How to give: Usually give every six hours around the clock. Can be given every eight hours in a mild case or if symptoms have improved greatly. Sometimes is used less frequently.

Dosage: We give liquid or tablets in a dose of 0.5 milligrams per kilogram per dose every six hours to start. We adjust dose depending on the child's progress and the medication's side effects. The usual starting dose is:

22 pound child - 5 mg (2.5cc) every six hours
44 pound child - 10 mg (5.0cc) every six hours

Comments: We rarely use beta-adrenergic drugs by mouth in children over three years of age. These children can achieve the same benefit at a fraction of the dose by using the inhaled form of the drug. Side effects are considerably less.

Albuterol
Brand names: Proventil, Ventolin

Metaproterenol
Brand names: Alupent, Metaprel

Indications:
- prevent bronchoconstriction due to exercise, cold and other triggers
- get relief while theophylline is building up at the beginning of an attack
- treat minor episodes of wheezing
- relieve symptoms with sudden onset
- eliminate symptoms which are not controlled by standard dose of theophylline
- insure that airways are open prior to using cromolyn

Desired effect: Relaxes smooth muscle around the bronchial tubes and allows the tubes to open more

Side effects: Less than liquid or tablet since dose is smaller. Shakiness, rapid heart beat, nervousness, nausea, vomiting, pallor, cough.

Form: Inhaler   albuterol   0.090 mg/spray
                       metaproterenol   0.65 mg/spray

Time Factor: Begins to work in a minute with full effect in fifteen minutes. Effect should last four hours. If it doesn't your inhaler is dirty or empty, your technique is bad or your asthma is out of control and you should consult your physician.

How to give: A double whiff two minutes apart is the standard dose.

Dosage: A double whiff every four hours while awake as needed up to five times a day. A double whiff of albuterol will provide somewhat greater effect and last somewhat longer than a double whiff of metaproterenol.

Comments: Inhaler must be used correctly or it will provide little benefit. Technique should be reviewed at every doctor's visit until it is perfect. After that review every six months is adequate. Always bring your inhaler when you visit the doctor.

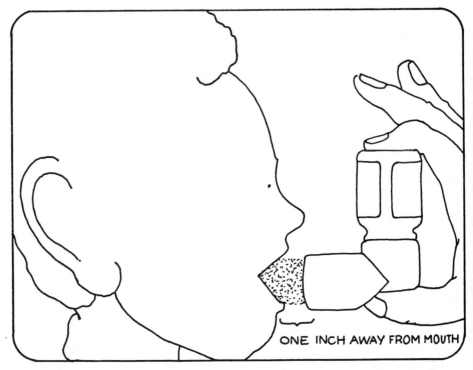

ONE INCH AWAY FROM MOUTH

PROPER INHALER POSITION

INSTRUCTIONS FOR USE OF INHALER
(metaproterenol or albuterol)

1. Put mouthpiece on cannister.
2. Stand up.
3. Shake inhaler for two seconds.
4. Position inhaler with cannister above mouthpiece (upside down).
5. Hold mouthpiece one inch from lips and open mouth wide. This position allows you to:
   - point the inhaler properly toward the back of your throat
   - draw the medicine into your mouth in a steady stream
   - have another person check to see that you are really pulling the medicine in

   Putting your lips around the mouthpiece as directed in the package instructions may prevent you from getting the full dose because:
   - *the mouthpiece may be misdirected*
   - *much of the medicine hits the cheeks and palate because of turbulence on release*
   - *no one can check to see that your timing is right.*
6. Breathe naturally, then
7. Open mouth wide and begin to inhale.
8. Squeeze cannister on mouthpiece and take about <u>two seconds</u> to inhale as deeply as you can.
9. Hold your breath for as long as you can up to <u>ten seconds</u>.
10. Keep your mouth open. If medicine floats out of your mouth, it didn't get deep enough. It is safe to repeat the dose without counting this one.
11. Wait <u>two minutes.</u>
12. Repeat steps 2 through 9. Most people benefit from a second inhalation. It delivers medicine into the windpipes that have been opened by the first whiff.
    - You should feel better five minutes after using inhaler.
    - The effect lasts for about four hours.
    - Do not use more than five double whiffs a day unless you check with your doctor.
    - A person who needs the inhaler more often may be going out of control. S/He should be checked to see if changes should be made in other medications.

Much of this information comes from an article by T.B. Harper, and R.C. Strunk, "Techniques of administration of metered-dose aerosolized drugs in asthmatic children." published in the <u>American Journal of Disease of Childhood</u>, Volume 135, pages 218-221, 1981.

CHECK LIST FOR MONITORING INHALER USE

We give our patients written and verbal instructions and demonstration before they use the inhaler the first time. We observe the patient's technique and correct defects before s/he fills his prescription. At the beginning of the next visit s/he is asked to demonstrate its use. When I reviewed technique at a followup visit for twenty consecutive patients I found that hardly anyone used the inhaler properly. So I designed a check list for home use. We now try to review inhaler use each time the patient visits the office for any reason. Technique has improved and patients note that the effect of the inhaler lasts longer.

*   *   *

Check each line while watching inhaler technique. Sheet can be used for several trials.

_____ stand up

_____ shake inhaler two seconds

_____ cannister above mouthpiece

_____ mouthpiece one inch from mouth

_____ breathe naturally

_____ open mouth wide and inhale to limit

_____ keep mouth open

_____ hold breath as long as you can up to ten seconds

Common mistakes are:
- inhalation is too fast. This leads to deposition of medicine on the palate instead of in the windpipes.
- exhaling too soon. Medication leaves the windpipes before it can settle where it is needed.
- necessity for a second inhalation is forgotten. Medication is not delivered to the newly expanded windpipes.
- interval between whiffs is less than two minutes. Medicine does not reach destination.

Your doctor can get a practice inhaler for you. Since it contains propellant but no medicine you can practice several times without getting shaky. Timing is the biggest problem. Many people find it hard to pull air in at the exact time to release the medicine. Breathing in slowly just before you squeeze may help you take the deep inspiration at the right time.

*   *   *

A mother told me she was concerned about her eleven-year-old hockey-playing son. He had to come off the ice three times in three weeks because of wheezing. This had not happened before. He ordinarily used an inhaler before practice and games. She did not think he was getting any benefit from his inhaler these days. I asked when he had cleaned it last. She didn't know since that was his responsibility. Well, all it took was a little soap and water and he was back to his usual game.

*   *   *

A ten-year-old boy with mild asthma uses an inhaler as his sole medication to control wheezing. He mentioned that he was using it at bedtime but awakened with wheezing in the middle of the night and had to use it again. Not terrific. His asthma wasn't bad enough to cause that much trouble. On reviewing his inhaler technique, I found that he only used a single whiff. When he changed to a double whiff, he was able to sleep through the night.

*   *   *

Father with asthma, "Thanks for teaching me to use the inhaler. Both my son and I are doing a lot better. I switched from the technique on the package insert to the instructions in CHILDREN WITH ASTHMA and now get more complete and sustained relief.

INHALATION DEVICES

We prescribe inhaled beta-adrenergic drugs for three quarters of the more than four hundred children with asthma in our practice. It is impossible for infants to use a metered dose inhaler (MDI). Young children (three to seven years) have great difficulty with timing inhalation to match delivery of the puff from the inhaler. The bad taste of the medication accentuates this problem. Children eight and older also have trouble with timing.

Powered Nebulizer:

Over the past year we have prescribed a number of these air compressors for children under three years of age. They are useful for delivering beta-adrenergic drugs directly to the airway of patients who are too young to use an inhaler. The cost, $115-200, is a small price to pay to keep a child out of the emergency room or the hospital. Make sure you check prices as they vary greatly for the same machine. I believe a powered nebulizer should be in the home of every child under three years old who has been hospitalized for asthma. Pulmo-Aide, available from Devilbiss Company, Somerset, Pennsylvania, 15501, Medi-Mist, sold by Mountain Medical Equipment, Littleton, Colorado, and Maxi-Myst from the Mead Johnson Company, Evansville, Indiana, 47721 are the three most commonly used brands. Requires a prescription.

Bubble Reservoir:

Most three year olds can use this inexpensive device with a metered dose inhaler (MDI) after only minutes of practice. A large volume plastic reservoir holds the medication spray until the child is ready to breathe in. This eliminates the need for exact coordination required by the MDI. The reservoir (bubble) also dilutes the unpleasant taste of medication. An additional feature is an incentive marker which indicates adquate inspiration. It can be used with good effect in a mild or moderate attack. (INHAL-AID, available from Key Pharmaceuticals, Miami, Florida. Cost: about $15-20. Requires prescription.)

Tube:

Children over eight who have difficulty with timing the release of medications from a MDI with their inhalation will find a tube reservoir helpful. The simplest version of this is a piece of typing paper rolled to a tube eight inches long and two inches in diameter. The puff of medication is held in the tube until the patient inhales. Must inhale within 2-3 seconds and hold breath for ten seconds. The commercial version of the tube has a valve which prevents accidental exhalation of the medication. For best effect the inhalation must be held ten seconds rather than five to ten as stated on the device. Aero-Chamber. Available from Monaghan Medical Corporation, Plattsburgh, New York, 12901. Cost: $12-14.

MICHELLE AND THE BUBBLE

By Lynn Arseneau

My three-year-old daughter, Michelle, has had asthma since age one. She uses medications continuously, makes many trips to the pediatrician and emergency room and was hospitalized twice this year. Last fall I heard that we could control her attacks by giving her medication through a metered dose inhaler. The inhaler would take the place of an office visit for an injection of adrenalin and might prevent admission to the hospital. It would bring her breathing under control and make her attacks less traumatic for everyone.

We bought an inhaler and practiced the routine on the package insert so we would know how to use it when an attack came. The first time she needed the inhaler, we were visiting my father's farm. The whole family had been looking forward to this weekend of fun and relaxation. Michelle was playing outside when she began having difficulty breathing. She was wheezing and really pulling hard for air. For once I wasn't concerned. I knew the inhaler would save the weekend.

You can probably guess what took place next. My three-year-old started wheezing and was having trouble just trying to take a breath when along comes Mommy with these instructions: "O.K., honey, just stand up, open your mouth wide . . . I'll hold this thing in front of your mouth, blow out, now I'll spray, you inhale . . . in a steady stream, hold your breath now, 1-2-3-4-5-6-7-8-9-10. O.K., one more time. . . ."

FORGET IT! The spray goes everywhere but down her throat. Some has hit her tongue so she now knows how horrible it tastes. She refuses to try it a second time. Now our child who couldn't breathe is crying, upset and exhausted. Her mother is also crying, upset and exhausted! We head for home, call the doctor, take Michelle in for a long doctor's visit and injections. The weekend is ruined.

If I had known about the "Bubble," this scene could have been avoided. The Bubble is a plastic chamber which holds the inhaler spray and allows Michelle to breathe as often as necessary to inhale the spray. She doesn't need exact timing to get the medication into her windpipe. Because the medication is dispersed into a chamber full of air it is diluted and there is no bad taste. That really helps!

Even if she can only manage small breaths, the first few will allow enough medication through the airway and into the bronchioles to open these tubes so that the next breaths are deeper. I have noticed this by watching the incentive indicator that is attached to the mouthpiece. The incentive indicator is a hollow tube with a small plastic "float" inside. The float rises up with each inhalation. The deeper the inhalation, the higher the float rises.

Michelle finds the Bubble very easy to use. I know she is getting the full benefit of the medication and I also feel more in control. A treatment takes only four minutes and the incentive indicator is wonderful. My family is convinced that the Bubble has saved us a lot of difficulty. We don't leave home without it.

STEROIDS (Corticosteroids)
Emlen Jones, M.D.

Prednisone
Brand Name: Colisone, Deltasone, Meticorten, Orasone, Sterapred, Winpred

Indications:

Short term use:
- severe asthma attack which is not improving with usual theophylline and beta-adrenergic treatment.
- attack which occurs in patient who is already taking maximum doses of theophylline and/or cromolyn and a beta adrenergic drug.
- hospital treatment of almost all patients with asthma.

Long term use:
- treatment of patient whose symptoms cannot be controlled with aggressive use of theophylline, beta adrenergics, environmental control, cromolyn and allergy shots. Any child who requires short term oral steroids repeatedly probably needs long term steroid treatment.

Desired effects (These are all unique to steroids):

- Decrease swelling of cells lining the bronchioles.
- Decrease mucous production by cells lining the bronchioles.
- Restore responsiveness of bronchioles to beta-adrenergic drugs.

Side effects:

- rarely a problem if treatment lasts less than two weeks.
- two-four weeks: increased appetite, weight gain, feeling of well-being.
- more than four weeks of daily use:

    - suppresses body's other responses
    - inhibits growth
    - increase susceptibility to serious infections
    - cataract formation, acne, stretch marks on the skin, thinning of skin, increase in body hair, fluid accumulation in the skin, facial puffiness, headache, mood changes, increased urination and trouble sleeping, high blood pressure.

Precautions apply to long-term use:
- Tuberculosis test, chest x-ray must be done before use.
- Live virus vaccines (measles, mumps, rubella, polio and smallpox) must not be given.
- Increase dose with surgery or other stress (burns or serious illness) to make up for blunted stress response for up to a year after steroids stopped.
- Do not discontinue abruptly. Dose must be tapered.
- (No special care is needed when child gets a common illness like a cold, bronchitis, ear infection, pneumonia or urinary tract infection.)

Form: oral tablet; inhaled (see beclomethasone); intravenous.

Time factors: Effect seen in 8-24 hours.

Dosage: Prednisone: about one mg per pound for short term use. Given four times a day with food to prevent stomach irritation. Much lower dose for long-term use. Can be discontinued abruptly if given for less than three weeks. Burst of three to seven days avoids side effects.

Comments: Steroids are used to treat asthma when other medications will not work. They are also used for brief periods of instability. They are the last medications used for long-term maintenance. Serious side effects may occur with careless or prolonged use. Steroids are a synthetic form of a hormone that is naturally produced by the body's adrenal gland and which has an important function in the body's response to stress. In asthma the doses used are many fold greater than the body's normal levels.

Must wear a medical alert bracelet for one year after taking steroids daily for more than four weeks. This tells people that extra steroids must be given in case of serious accident or unusual stress. Legend should read: "Steroid dependent asthma - adrenal suppression."

*   *   *

Beclomethasone
Brand Name: Beclovent, Vanceril

Indications:

Many asthma experts find this a helpful drug for certain children who require long term treatment with steroids. Consult your physician for specific indications and dosage.

CROMOLYN SODIUM

Brand Name: Intal

Indications:
- asthma which requires daily medication. Cromolyn may help 60-80% of these children.
- theophylline not effective or not well tolerated.
- exercise induced asthma.
- episodic exposure to animal dander such as cat or dog.

Desired effect: Prevents release of substances within the bronchiole which cause bronchospasm.

Side effects: occur much less often than with the other drugs used to treat asthma.
- throat irritation, bad taste in mouth, rare allergic reaction, wheeze.

Form and Dose:
- Powder-filled capsule. Inhaled using a special propeller inhaler (Spinhaler). One capsule is inhaled four times a day, regardless of age. Fifty percent of patients can reduce the dose to three times daily after an initial period of one or two months. Occasionally two doses a day are effective.
- Nebulized solution: Infants and children can take cromolyn as a nebulized solution by means of a powered nebulizer (see p. 66). It is usually given simultaneously with a beta-adrenergic.

Time factors:
- four to eight weeks of treatment are often required before full effect is seen.
- thirty minutes before exposure to allergen (for example, cat) to prevent or reduce wheezing on a single exposure. Better yet, it can be used four times both the day before and on the day of the planned exposure.
- fifteen minutes before exercise to prevent exercise-induced asthma. Often used following beta-adrenergic drug when neither cromolyn or the beta-adrenergic provide adequate protection.

Comments:

- The windpipes must be open for cromolyn to be effective. Before starting treatment the physician must demonstrate that the windpipes are open by doing pulmonary function tests. If pulmonary function is not normal the patient must be treated aggressively and cleared before cromolyn is started or the drug will not be effective.
- To insure an open airway and to prevent a cough during administration many patients take two inhalations of a beta-adrenergic drug before inhaling cromolyn.
- The occasional older child or teenager who can not control a cough when inhaling cromolyn powder will usually tolerate the nebulized solution.
- Use of cromolyn may allow decrease or elimination of daily theophylline dose in cases of perennial asthma.
- Cromolyn is not helpful in treating an asthma attack. However its use should be continued during an attack unless it provokes coughing.
- Directions for use supplied in the package insert are excellent.

COMBINATION DRUGS

In the past theophylline was often prescribed in combination with ephedrine (an adrenergic drug) and either a sedative or a tranquillizer. Most asthma experts now strongly oppose the use of three drugs in one syrup or tablet. As you know, it is difficult enough to figure out how much of a single medication your child needs at a particular time. Rational treatment of asthma calls for the increase of a single medication to the point at which the patient either gets better or gets unacceptable side effects from the medication. Additional drugs are added as needed. With fixed drug combinations one often gets side effects from one ingredient before getting adequate benefit from another.

GENERAL INSTRUCTIONS

Instructions for the management of an asthma attack are too complicated to be given only orally. There are many opportunities for errors, both by the physician and by the parent. Medicine with a single name may come in several strengths and dosage forms. Often a child must take several medications simulaneously.

This preprinted form allows the physician to provide individualized directions for the parent in an efficient manner. It gives parents the opportunity to look at the instructions and ask questions about them in the office. It eliminates the need for guesswork in recall after they leave the office.

GENERAL INSTRUCTIONS FOR TREATING
AN ASTHMA ATTACK

_____ is being treated for asthma.

It is of _____ severity.

__ An attack usually comes on after exercise, in cold weather, with an infection, or at an unpredictable time.

__ Theophylline as _____ mg every ____ hours.

__ It should be continued for _____ days after the symptoms stop.

__ Since it usually takes thirteen hours before this medicine reaches effective levels, s/he should take _____ mg of plain theophylline with the first dose.

__ S/He should use the a beta-adrenergic inhaler one double whiff every four hours while awake for the first day and then up to four times a day if still wheezing.

__ If s/he is not greatly improved after 24 hours of treatment, please contact one of the pediatricians.

__ While taking medication for an asthma attack, s/he should drink at least ____ ounces of liquid a day.

20 lbs - 22; 30 lbs - 34; 40 lbs - 40; 60 lbs - 54; 80 lbs - 64; 150 lbs - 80 (Based on 1500 cc/square meter of body surface area)

__ Prednisone _____ 5 milligram tablets at 9 am, 1 pm, 5 pm, and 9 pm, daily for _____ days.

__ Continue taking cromolyn unless it causes coughing.

__ The beta-adrenergic inhaler should be used 15 minutes before strenuous exercise to prevent wheezing. The effects usually lasts four hours.

__ Please check your handouts for side effects of medication.

__ Call the office if you have any questions or think the doctor or pharmicist made an error.

_____, M.D.

MATT

Some Principles for Managing Asthma

by Joe Duffy

I have the distinct advantage of writing this narrative about a year and a half after reading my wife's story of our son, Matthew. Since there's little to be gained from repeating the history and anecdotes as told by Jeamie, I'll simply try to supplement it from a somewhat different, and more general, perspective.

Matthew is eight years old now and is a happy, healthy, outgoing, well-adjusted, athletic child with budding interests in rock'n roll, fast cars, baseball, and junk food. Until maybe a year ago, however, if someone asked "How's Matt?", the status of his asthma would probably have emerged early in the answer and received considerable emphasis. In fact, the qualities I just described--the qualities that represent what Matt really is--sometimes were never mentioned or were given only token attention. Today, asthma often is not part of the answer at all to "how's Matt?" unless the question is rephrased to "how's his asthma?" Today, the short answer to that question usually is "good."

What was involved in this change from Matt's asthma being a dominant influence on our family to its fitting rather easily into the background of our daily routines? Probably a number of things have been important. I'll try to review those which seem most important to me, and which I believe may be of near universal importance to families with a child who has moderately severe asthma.

First, Jeamie and I have become good observers of behaviors which signal that Matt's asthma is active to a degree that requires close watching, an increase or change in medication, or a call or visit to his doctor. The importance of being good observers of these behaviors stems from our understanding that the best way to treat asthma is to control it in a way that prevents it from becoming active. When it becomes active one must treat it aggressively enough to restore breathing function to "normal" or keep it in check until the triggering event (cold, weather, allergen, etc.) is no longer present. Arriving at this understanding was of major importance in our adjustment to and treatment of Matt's asthma. When Matt was one to three years old, I very often reacted to the beginning of an asthma episode with a kind of denial. I attributed his wheezing or coughing to a cold or some other cause and assumed that they would simply not last or worsen. This attitude often served to delay treatment and, on occasion, resulted in the episode becoming worse than it needed to be. Today, we're good at recognizing when symptoms or behavior are asthma related. When they are we actively manage the problem as early as possible.

The second factor is strongly related to the first. Jeamie and I have learned as much about asthma as is necessary for us to play an active role in its management. We do not accept the notion that the physician is the only person capable of accurately observing and managing asthma in childhood. We believe that the parents and the patient are almost always in a better position to observe the onset and progression of symptoms and the effect of treatment, long before and long after the physician has examined the child. We have been extremely fortunate to have pediatricians whose philosophy of asthma treatment strongly involves the parents' becoming active in treatment.

It often is necessary to let the physician know that you wish to participate and convince him/her that you are capable of doing so. Parents must realize that asthma may be managed with maximum benefit when the physician is not expected to play an independent, omnipotent god. The physician should feel comfortable enough with the parents' interest and motivation to participate that it is not necessary--for effective management or his/her ego--to play god. The physician thus becomes the knowledge source about asthma and the primary organizer of management. The parents (and child) become aides who contribute importantly to the collection of diagnostic information and are able to arrive independently and reliably at logical decisions about certain aspects of management. These include increase or decrease in medication, addition of stronger medication on hand, and simply knowing when to call the doctor.

Under this philosophy of management, a lot of work is required. This "work," for us, has included: reading and learning facts about the nature of asthma; learning what its symptoms are; learning how to reliably recognize those symptoms and their meaning; learning about the purpose of medications and their intended results and negative side effects; learning about the purpose and meaning of measuring blood levels for theophylline; learning to estimate I/O ratios and breathing rates; getting a feel--over time--for how to report relevant facts to the physician or nurse; and, perhaps most importantly, learning how to ask questions--without embarrassment--that will contribute to future management of the problem. This has not been easy, but it hasn't been too hard either. It has taken years but the results have been rewarding. For us, in managing Matt's asthma, knowledge is not only power, but also the source for reducing anxiety and fear about a problem which need not be the unknowable monster many people perceive it to be.

The last factor which has been important in managing Matt's asthma deals with our relationship with him. We have tried our best to mark our relationship with calmness, confidence, honesty, education, and an absence of rewards for being sick. Calmness and confidence are strongly tied to one another. We're able to be calm during asthma episodes (even those necessitating hospitalization) because of the factors I mentioned previously: calm because we recognize his symptoms and their meaning, and calm because we understand the reasons for the treatment he receives. This "knowledge as power" translates into confidence when interacting with Matt during an asthma episode. We're able to tell him why we're asking certain questions ("Do you feel wheezy?") or observing his breathing rate, or listening for wheezing. We can tell him what and why we're doing the things we find necessary to manage the problem (increase medication or fluid intake, visit the doctor, or go to the hospital). I know the ability to be calm and confident makes Jeamie and me feel good about ourselves at such times. I'm sure our calmness and confidence reduce any "fear of the unknown" that Matt might have, and minimize the role that anxiety might play in increasing the severity of an episode. We've really begun to see the payoff of this approach in the last two years--Matt is now at least as calm as we are during an episode.

We've also learned that honesty and education about the problem really pay off in terms of Matt's realism and calmness about his asthma. For example, if we need to see a doctor during an episode, we tell him he may have to have a shot and that it will hurt a bit--in fact, shots are amazingly routine now because he gets two allergy shots every Friday. When hospitalization has been necessary we've told him that we are going before we got there, why, and what would be done when we arrive--the last time he was hospitalized, he told us what probably would be done, and he was right! To the best of our ability, we also answer any question he asks, such as: Why do I have asthma? Will I always get allergy shots? Will I always have asthma? What does this pill do? When we can't answer a question, he is encouraged to ask his doctor or nurse when he sees them next.

Finally, we've tried to avoid rewarding Matt for having asthma. Early in Matt's history we occasionally found ourselves offering "treats" in association with asthma episodes. For example, ice cream after a shot or a new toy immediately after entering the hospital. These rewards were given out of love and concern (sometimes relief!), but the risk run is that the child may learn to associate tangible rewards, attention, and affection with having asthma. The pros call this "secondary gain," which means the child may "learn," very subtly, that asthma has its benefits and rewards. The ultimate danger is that this could lead to the start, maintenance, or worsening of an episode when it otherwise would not have occurred in order to get the desired payoffs. Asthma may be used as an excuse for not doing things which can and should be done (going to school, helping around the house, exercising). We've tried to combat this in several ways. We postpone "treats" until Matt's episode has passed and reward him for doing well at "getting better." For example, we once gave him a toy he wanted after he came home from the hospital, not while he was in the hospital. We told him it was for being so cooperative and good while he was there, which probably shortened his stay. We place a minimum of restrictions on his physical activities, even when he is wheezy. The exceptions to this involve avoidance of known major allergens for Matt. For example, he can't go to a barn down the road because he's very allergic to the horses there. We've discovered that Matt has always been a good judge of what he should and shouldn't do physically. If he's quite wheezy and plays soccer, he'll often quit in just a short time. We always try to encourage physical and athletic activity, but balance it by acknowledging his good common sense to quit when it's appropriate. Third, we've tried to minimize the attention we pay to his asthma during our daily routines: medicine gets put on the table to be taken, not talked about; allergy shots are an in-and-out-of-the-doctor's-office-as-fast-as-possible event. Asthma is a topic of conversation only if Matt raises the issue.

I think all of these things have helped us and Matt to think of him, not as "an asthmatic" but as a youngster who just happens to have asthma, just like other people have warts, colds, arthritis, and hemmorhoids. It's a part of what he is, and it deserves a degree of attention. But it's only a small part and, hopefully, not very important to how people view him nor to his ultimate achievements.

Before closing, I should admit to recognizing that this narrative has been somewhat idealistic and simplistic. Our present attitudes and beliefs about Matt's asthma are colored by the relatively long period of time in which we have not had to deal with major episodes and also by our nearly eight years of experience with the problem. In addition, many of the things I've said we do, or have done, which are good we don't always do or find very difficult to do. On the other hand, I do believe we've learned to deal with Matt's asthma effectively and feel confident that the factors discussed above are a good part of the reason why.

ASTHMA QUIZ

NAME: _____

1. Name three changes in the windpipe caused by asthma.

   _____

   _____

   _____

2. Name one early clue your child shows before he starts an asthma attack.

   _____

3. Name one event which triggers asthma in your child.

   _____

4. Why should you give medication to prevent an asthma attack?

   _____

5. Why should you give medication early to treat an attack?

   _____

6. What are the four most important things to monitor in an asthma attack?

   _____   _____

   _____   _____

7. How long should your child take medicine for an asthma attack?

   _____

8. How much liquid should your child drink in 24 hours with an asthma attack?

   _____

9. Under what circumstances should the blood theophylline level be checked?

_____

10. Beta-adrenergic inhaler (Alupent, Metaprel, Ventolin, Proventil): Please answer true or false.

   a. Must breathe in as deeply as possible ____

   b. Must hold breath for ten seconds ____

   c. Must always take a double whiff, unless doctor says otherwise ____

   d. Must have two-minute interval between whiffs ____

   e. Inhaler can prevent wheezing which is set off by exercise ____

   f. More effective if used when standing up because one can take deeper breaths ____

   g. Must clean plastic mouthpiece with warm water when see dirt or film ____

11. What medication does your child take?

Name	Strength mg	Action*	Time to Reach Full Effect	Effect Lasts

* 1. dilates windpipe, 2. reduces swelling,   3. reduces mucus, 4. prevents attacks, 5. prevents exercise-induced asthma.

ASTHMA QUIZ: ANSWERS

NAME: _____

1. Name three changes in the windpipe caused by asthma.

   muscles around the bronchioles tighten up

   cells lining the windpipe swell

   mucus is produced by cells inside windpipe

2. Name one early clue your child shows before he starts an asthma attack.

   coughs, sneezes, watery eyes, chest gets tight, gets upset,

   other

3. Name one event which triggers asthma in your child.

   infection, exercise, cold, weather change, pollutant, laugh

4. Why should you give medication to prevent an asthma attack?

   It is easier to prevent an attack than to treat it. The three

   responses in the windpipe haven't started.

5. Why should you give medication early to treat an attack?

   Medication works better before swelling and mucus become

   severe. It only takes minutes to relax tight bronchiole

   muscles but days to clear up swelling and mucus.

6. What are the four most important things to monitor in an asthma attack?

I:O ratio	retractions
wheezing	respiratory rate

7. How long should your child take medicine for an asthma attack?

For two days after all symptoms stop unless doctor says otherwise.

8. How much liquid should your child drink in 24 hours with an asthma attack?

20 lbs-22 oz, 30 lbs-30 oz, 40 lbs-40 oz, 60 lbs-50 oz, 80 lbs-56oz, 150 lbs-80 oz

9. Under what circumstances should the blood theophylline level be checked?

Before increasing dose above 20 mg/kg

if any concern about toxicity.

10. Beta-adrenergic inhaler (Alupent, Metaprel, Ventolin, Proventil): Please answer true or false.

   a. Must breathe in as deeply as possible true

   b. Must hold breath for ten seconds true

   c. Must always take a double whiff, unless doctor says otherwise true

   d. Must have two-minute interval between whiffs true

   e. Inhaler can prevent wheezing which is set off by exercise true

   f. More effective if used when standing up because one can take deeper breaths true

   g. Must clean plastic mouthpiece with soap and warm water when see dirt or film true

11. What medication does your child take?

Name	Strength mg	Action*	Time to Reach Full Effect	Effect Lasts
Theodur tablets	100,200,300	1	13 hrs	12 hrs
Theodur sprinkles	50, 75, 125, 200	1	13 hrs	12 hrs
Slophyllin Gyrocaps	60, 125, 250	1	10 hrs	8 hrs
Theophyllin tablet	100, 200, 300	1	2 hrs	6 hrs
Theophyllin liquid	varies	1	1 hr	6 hrs
Alupent liquid	10, 20	1	30 min	6 hrs
Beta-adrenergic		1	1-15 min	4 hrs
Prednisone	5	2, 3	16 hrs	36 hrs
Cromolyn	20	4	4 wks	days
		5	15 min	4 hrs

* 1. dilates windpipe, 2. reduces swelling, 3. reduces mucus, 4. prevents attacks, 5. prevents exercise-induced asthma.

Chapter Four
GETTING IT TOGETHER

"Helping Parents Manage Asthma" describes our experience in helping parents attain mastery over this disruptive illness. In the parents' asthma group they integrate information and make contact with parents facing similar problems. "Feelings" summarizes a sentence composition exercise. Four parents briefly relate their experiences with asthma. "Instructions for Babysitters" rounds out the chapter.

I want to discuss what happens in the physician's office, what takes place in our parents' education and support group, and what happens at home. First, I would like to say something about the language we use and the goals we set. We refer to our patients as children first, and mention their problem second.

We do not use the word "asthmatic" as a noun. We feel this term describes the child in terms of a problem and thus distorts the attitudes of parents, physicians, teachers and friends toward the child. By saying 'child with asthma' we indicate that the child is generally healthy, yet has a problem which requires care.

We assume and expect that each one of our patients with asthma will be able to carry out every activity which is usual for his or her age with rare exceptions. If they want to play hockey, run cross-country or compete in swimming, we encourage them to try. In fact, our patients take part in each of these activities. We do not make assumptions based on the child's past history. Just because a seven-year-old had been hospitalized 32 times for asthma before coming under our care does not mean that we will hospitalize him. We do not write excuses to get a child out of gym because of wheezing...unless we have tried every other means to prevent or control it.

In the case of any chronic illness, we believe the parent should act as a physician and the physician should serve as a consultant. The parent observes the child's symptoms and physical state. S/He makes management decisions within certain limits set by the physician consultant. We expect parents to be active participants in the care of their child's problem. We do our best to support them, providing easy access to the office, 24-hour access to the physician in case of serious problems, and the encouragement to manage the child's problem at home to the best of their ability. Parents grow in their ability to care for their child with asthma as they learn more about it in office visits, from our parents' group, from their reading, from experiences with their child, and from conversation with parents of other children who have asthma.

When I came to Amherst in 1977, I found that asthma was the most common chronic illness facing my patients. In only a few of these children was this problem controlled adequately. Parents had little understanding of asthma or the functions of the various medications used to treat it. Now, parents can't treat asthma unless they can recognize an attack. They can't regulate medication dosage unless they know the functions and side effects of various drugs used to treat it.

In my first year in Amherst, I cared for more than forty children with asthma. Many of them had not been previously diagnosed as having asthma. You may have heard that asthma is the most underdiagnosed and undertreated chronic illness in children. Well, it's true! Initially, I found that I was spending a lot of time trying to describe the workings of asthma to parents. I also discussed medications, their desired effects, and their toxicity. After a few months, I started writing handouts covering these subjects to save time, to give parents something to refer to, and to reduce the cost of the visit to the patient.

My goal is to help parents change their behavior so they can care for their child's problem with competence and confidence. It takes several steps to change behavior: first a person must acquire knowledge, a basic understanding of what is going on. Second, one must develop skill in using this new knowledge. This takes practice and supervision. Third, one must develop an attitude which enables one to treat asthma at home. Finally, the behavior change must be supported in order to be sustained.

At the first visit for an attack of wheezing, I give the parent three handouts. The first sheet is entitled, "Judging the Severity of an Asthma Attack" (see Chapter 2). Parents have a dilemma. They want to provide decent medical care for their children, but also have to conserve their time and money. Some of our patients live 25 miles from the office, so they must learn when to come in for help and when to handle an attack themselves. They don't want to come in too early, but if they wait too long an episode will be more difficult to treat. My partner, Emlen Jones, developed this handout. In it, he describes the major factors to observe in assessing the severity of an attack. We concentrate on the ratio of breathing in (inspiration) to breathing out (expiration). After the parent has read this description in the office, I ask her/him to breathe with me and to get the feel of the time which expiration contributes to the breathing cycle. As I vary my breathing, the parent begins to catch on. We practice this at later visits until the parent can make an accurate judgment of the inspiratory to expiratory ratio.

The second sheet describes theophylline (see Chapter 3), a major drug used in the treatment of asthma. It covers the effects, indications, dose, duration and side effects of the drug. We discuss the factors which cause the amount and timing of a dosage to vary. We expect parents to know their child's daily dosage and how to vary it with the severity of symptoms. They should be able to tell whether the doctor made an error in writing the prescription or if the druggist made a mistake in filling it. This has actually happened on several occasions. We give general information and instructions in printed form and encourage parents or patients to write down specific instructions about medication during the office visit. It would be impossible for anyone to remember all this information if it were only provided verbally.

At the same visit I point out what a retraction is and how it decreases with treatment. Finally we discuss the cause and significance of wheezing. In a few minutes of instruction the parent gains the knowledge to judge the severity of an attack. In the future this parent will be able to detect signs of improvement or worsening after giving medication and will be able to decide whether a visit or call to the doctor is necessary. S/He also acquires the vocabulary needed to communicate clearly with the physician by phone.

The third sheet is the "Asthma Record" (see Chapter 2). It is the keystone of our program of education for parents and children in managing asthma. Early on we wasted most of each visit in trying to recall the effects of colds, activity and medication on symptoms. To save time, I devised this record for the parent or older child to record symptoms and factors which influence them on a daily basis. This record gives the parent an opportunity to analyze what is going on even before s/he sees me. The parent will often suggest a change in medication based on her/his observations. If s/he misses a clue, I can pick it up. In addition, I can tell if the medication is being used in the right amount and at the proper intervals.

If the child is moderately ill with the first asthma attack we stay in contact by phone and I schedule a follow-up visit for a week later. At this time I answer parents' questions about medications and asthma, review the asthma record and how to assess the severity of an attack. I also urge the parent to buy the book by Guy Parcel, Teaching Myself About Asthma (see Chapter 6). This book is a jewel! It is written at a third grade reading level and thus can be studied by parent and child together. It does an excellent job of describing breathing, as well as the triggers, early clues, and progress of an asthma attack.

Knowledge and skill are not enough. The parent must develop an attitude which allows her/him to try the new behaviors. Many parents are frightened by an attack, afraid that their child may die if not rushed to the doctor immediately. Our parents' education/support group has changed parents' attitudes in a dramatic way. Let me tell you about it.

Five years ago, I started the first group with the help of Sharon Dorfman, a health educator in our office. The goals of the program are:

-- to increase parents' knowledge of facts and myths about asthma, its treatment and the prevention of attacks.
-- to provide a comfortable setting for sharing feelings about the ways in which asthma affects the child, parents and others.
-- to build the family's skills in monitoring the child with asthma, recognizing the onset of "attacks" and making appropriate decisions about using medications, contacting practitioners, dealing with schools, friends and babysitters.

A great deal of information is presented at the first session. Much of it has been covered with parents at office visits. However, reviewing this with eight to 12 other parents who are at various stages of dealing with the same problem is a great help. This is the first time some parents see that others are dealing with the same problems that they are struggling with day-to-day. In the second session, we use a sentence completion exercise to bring out prevailing attitudes of fear, anger, guilt and pessimism which exist in the parents of children with a chronic illness. Once in the open, these feelings can be discussed and related to by all parents. We also work to create a positive attitude by demonstrating that parents can manage these various practical problems. Parents learn from each other how to cope with overnight visits, problems with teachers, dealing with doctors, and the fright of an acute attack. This learning among parents help them feel more independent of the doctor and thus more ready to handle problems on their own.

Once a parent has acquired the knowledge and skill to handle an attack, and has gone through some attitudinal changes, s/he is able to behave in an effective manner. S/He can treat an attack early, will know how to judge progress, and will be able to control asthma rather than letting it control her/him.

Optimal management is only possible when the parent gets support and guidance from the physician consultant. We ask the parent to bring the child to the office if s/he is unsure of her/his ability to judge the severity of an attack. At the visit, we compare the parent's observations and assessment with ours; that way, s/he can increase the knowledge and skill in dealing with asthma at each visit. We are available for consultation 24 hours a day every day of the year if a child with asthma has a serious problem. This means that our parents don't have to worry that their child will be cared for by an unknown physician in an unfamiliar way. With this kind of support, parents have learned to become confident managers of their children's asthma.

PARENTS' ASTHMA GROUP

During four hours crammed with information, demonstrations, practice and discussion, parents have an opportunity to consolidate their knowledge of asthma and its treatment. They discuss their feelings with parents who have had similar experiences. They find that their reactions to asthma and the disruptions it causes in their lives are shared by many others. Finally, it gives them a chance to get better acquainted, in a relaxed atmosphere, with the physicians who will take care of their child when s/he is having trouble.

After parents participate in the asthma group, they become more capable of monitoring their child's asthma and of handling attacks. Their increased knowledge and skills result in a more confident attitude and less need to restrict the child. The children increase their participation in sports and social interactions. The family as a whole functions better because the stress on it is reduced.

Some of these changes are illustrated by comments obtained from mothers three months after they attended the initial asthma group sessions in 1978.

"Feel more secure about treatment, can now call in when Matt has an attack and can change dose by phone with physician's help, based upon the report I give him."

"Feel more secure about medication, not worried about giving Mike an overdose and killing him. Feel more confident about when he should be seen by physician. Asthma, itself, is unchanged."

"Found out Lindsay's problem is not as severe as originally thought, compared to other children. Feel comfortable that doctor has studied asthma and knows a lot about it. Feel information before a crisis is worth its weight in gold. Able to anticipate and organize things."

"Much more comfortable with Josh's asthma. Recently he started wheezing at wilderness camp 100 miles away. The nurse called, frantic, at 7 a.m. and asked me to come and get him right away. I assessed the situation on the phone and gave instructions to the nurse for treatment. Josh remained at camp with his class. I was able to go to work."

INITIAL INFORMATION
Parents' Asthma Group

Goals: To increase parents' knowledge of the facts and myths about asthma, its treatment and the prevention of attacks.

To provide a comfortable setting for sharing feelings about the way in which asthma affects the child, parents and others.

To build the family's skills in monitoring the child with asthma, recognizing the onset of attacks and making appropriate decisions about using medications, contacting practitioners, and dealing with schools, friends and babysitters.

Who is invited: Parents of children with asthma who are patients at Amherst Medical Associates

Where and when: Two 2-hour sessions.
First session: 7:30 p.m. May 29, 1985
Second session: 7:30 p.m. June 5, 1985
Both sessions will be held in the Pediatric waiting room at Amherst Medical Associates. Individual consultations will be provided at the end of each session.

Since the second session builds on the learning and sharing of the first, only parents who attend the first meeting can participate in the second.

Preparation: We are counting on everyone to read Chapters 2 and 3 of CHILDREN WITH ASTHMA: A MANUAL FOR PARENTS before the first session so that we can have more time for discussion.

Fee: $40.00 per family for the series. Those with Valley Health Plan are already overed.

Staff: Drs. Thomas F. Plaut and Emlen H. Jones (second session).

For more information: Call the pediatric office at 253-XXXX and ask for one of the nursing staff.

Complete and return the enclosed registration form and the asthma visit questionnaire if you wish to attend.

REGISTRATION FORM
Parents' Asthma Group

If you decide to participate in the series, please complete this form and send it to AMA Pediatrics. Your thoughtful responses will help us plan a program that reflects the backgrounds, concerns and interests of group members.

How interested are you in learning about the following?

Please rate on a scale of 0 to 5--0 means "not at all"
5 means "strongly interested"

_____ asthma medications
_____ breathing exercises
_____ controlling the environment of a child with asthma
_____ early clues that an "attack" may be starting
_____ how asthma is diagnosed
_____ the effect of asthma on overall health
_____ the relationship to allergies
_____ the role of emotions
_____ things that may "trigger" an attack
_____ what happens in the body during an attack
_____ when to seek medical assistance
_____ others (please list) _____

Please feel free to add any other questions, interests or areas of concern related to asthma that you would like to suggest for inclusion in the series.

Name of Child: _____

Parents' Names: _____

_____

Phone Number   (Home) _____

(Work) _____

By registering early you reserve a place in the next Parents' Asthma Group. Once the dates are set we will contact you to confirm. At that time you will be asked to make a commitment to attend both sessions.

AGENDA
Parents' Asthma Group

First Session:

7:30 Get acquainted: Give your name, the name and age of your child, duration of his/her asthma, an asthma concern and make an unrelated comment.

7:40 Introduction: We have these sessions to help parents understand asthma so they can see that their child gets the proper treatment when s/he needs it.

7:50 Breathing: Chest and lung structure and function.

8:00 Asthma attack: Constriction of smooth muscle, swelling of windpipe lining, secretion of mucus.

8:10 Triggers: Infection, exercise, irritants, emotion, allergens.

8:20 Early clues: Important in deciding when to medicate.

8:30 Five minute stretch.

8:35 Recording: Helps in adjusting medication amount and duration.

8:45 Severity: Parents can judge accurately using wheezing, I:O ratio and retraction.

8:55 Medications: The two main drugs are theophylline and metaproterenol.

9:10 Questions

9:25 Evaluation sheet: Need this to plan next session.

9:30 Individual consultations.

Please Fill out feelings sheet and an asthma record on your child before the next meeting.

Second Session:

7:30 Environmental factors: house dust, mold, cigarette smoke.

7:40 Allergic factors: Triggers include animal dander, pollen and dust. Which child needs allergy evaluation?

7:50 Feelings: discussion will focus on the sentence completion exercise.

8:20 Prognosis: How serious is asthma? Who outgrows it?

8:25 Five minute stretch.

8:30 Other medications: steroids, cromolyn.

8:40 Peak flow meter: its use in office and home.

8:45 Instructions for parents. Information for school nurse, teacher and emergency room doctor.

8:55 Questions

9:25 Evaluation
Set date for three month follow-up meeting.

9:30 Individual consultations.

An asthma attack is always inconvenient and often disruptive. If you don't know how to take care of it, the attack can be very frightening, too. When your child has trouble breathing and you don't know what to do, you become anxious, excited and scared. Your distress has an unsettling effect on your child. The only thing you can think of is to get help as fast as possible.

Your child misses school. You have to miss work, in order to care for him or take him to the doctor. You feel you are not in control of events. You have less energy to spend on other members of the family. Plans go down the tube. You have to cancel or cut short family outings. Your child misses a basketball game or has to cancel an overnight visit.

Asthma is nobody's fault. You get angry that it happened to your family. There is nothing fair about asthma, diabetes, or a seizure disorder. Its occurrence is beyond a family's control. However, the outcome of an attack usually can be significantly affected by the family's knowledge, skill and attitude in managing the problem.

By the second session, the parents in the group have become acquainted with each other. A lot of discussion takes place during the sentence completion exercise on feelings. In a group of twelve parents, several will come up with the same words and phrases. My comments follow the parents' responses.

I think that having asthma makes my child feel...

-- like most other kids
-- haven't noticed a difference
-- different
-- different from other kids and often angry
-- frustrated that he cannot do everything he'd like to
-- frightened, anxious, tired
-- cautious

Between attacks some children are able to ignore their asthma completely. Other children have to be alert to triggers and early warning signs of an attack. This helps them to prevent some attacks and treat others early. A few children have asthma which is so severe that despite good management skills they get into difficulty.

Because of asthma, I think others treat my child differently by...

-- they don't
-- worry about medicine time only
-- letting him take a break when he is playing sports. Otherwise, others don't treat him differently.
-- wondering how it affects him
-- being overprotective
-- being nervous around her/him

It is hard to know how to deal with other people until you get your child's asthma straight in your own head. People who have a lot to do with your child - his playmates, hockey coach, teacher, baby sitter, friends' parents - should know enough about his asthma to deal with it in a relaxed fashion without being overprotective or demanding too much when he has an attack.

When my child has an asthma attack, I wish I was able to...

-- know why it's happening and judge the severity better
-- help him relax and have a well thought-out plan of action
-- feel sure about what I was doing right
-- console him, encourage him
-- breathe for him!
-- reverse it immediately

I suppose most of you have had each of these reactions.

I feel angry when...

-- I have to miss a lot of sleep because of his asthma
-- an attack interferes with family activities for a prolonged duration
-- I sit here and feel that I'm dumb and don't know enough about what's going to happen
-- he won't help himself until the attack gets more severe
-- he does not take his medication and I know he needs it
-- he "uses" his allergies and asthma for attention or as an excuse
-- he forgets his medicine at a friend's house
-- I can't do anything to help him

Asthma is not fair to parents. Sometimes you can do everything right yet an attack disrupts a family trip or forces you to leave work to care for your sick child. Asthma is not fair to children. They must be more responsible than their friends in monitoring their bodies and taking their medicines.

Because of asthma, I treat my child differently by...

-- I don't believe I do
-- encouraging him to learn methods to cope with asthma
-- I don't, except to check how she feels before she starts something strenuous
-- overprotecting sometimes, worrying about him more
-- not letting him play as hard
-- watching him too closely

Most parents in the asthma groups know when they are being overprotective of their children. This is a usual early reaction in caring for a child with asthma. As you gain understanding of asthma and your child's limits you can shift from overprotection to sensible management.

The aspect of my child's asthma that frightens me most is...

-- I don't feel frightened anymore, we understand how to handle it
-- there is none
-- he may not always be able to participate in any activity he wants
-- I won't know when or what to do
-- possible ill effects of long-term medication
-- the possibility of not reversing an attack
-- that the breathing would become so difficult he'd not be able to

Every parent whose child has severe asthma has worried about the child dying from an attack. Once they learn how to manage an attack, they worry much less. Actually, death from asthma is rare in childhood.

I feel guilty about...

-- I don't believe I do
-- not knowing enough when s/he has an attack
-- not detecting earliest signs
-- getting angry when he's sick
-- the fact that the asthma comes from my side of the family

In the past doctors thought asthma was caused by a defective mother-child relationship. We now know that there is no truth whatsoever in this theory. However, it is natural to feel some guilt. The important thing is not to dwell on it but rather to to learn more about asthma or how to interact better with your child.

When an asthma attack occurs, I think my child feels...

-- scared and angry that it's happening
-- frustrated - "What, again?"
-- unhappy and sometimes frightened
-- like sticking very close to mom and familiar surroundings
-- sick, is what he says

An asthma attack can be a scary, frustrating, disruptive, unhappy event. I never heard anyone say it was fun or even O.K.

During an attack, I become frightened when...

-- the medication is not bringing it under control and his breathing becomes more labored.
-- he coughs and can't keep his medicine down
-- she has to be hospitalized
-- he becomes gaunt, frightened
-- I think that I am losing control

All of this is frightening and it is time to call for help.

One would think that a parent's answers would depend primarily on the severity of his/her child's asthma. Actually, two other factors are of equal importance, the age of the child and the ability of the parents to manage an attack. Under age four, children often get into difficulty more quickly. Thus they are less likely to give their parents early warning.

Parents who have the knowledge and skill to manage an attack go through their routine without becoming anxious. They start treatment early and vigorously. They can judge when treatment is effective and do not worry unnecessarily. They know when an attack is getting worse despite aggressive treatment and contact the doctor for help before things get out of hand.

Another group of parents is clearly heard from in these comments. They know that they could be in control of the situation, but for some reason - perhaps not enough experience, study or planning - they are not able to perform well enough to manage a standard attack. One mother said she almost wished her son would have another attack soon so she could improve her skill in managing asthma at home.

Finally there is a group of parents who feel that they are not in control and don't see how they can be. Their presence in the parents' asthma group makes me believe that they will be able to learn to manage their child's asthma, as have dozens of families before them.

THE EFFECTS OF MIKE'S ASTHMA ON OUR FAMILY

By Kathy Bowler

The main effect is time. When Michael was young and frequently ill, he required a lot of time and attention quite often. I felt I could not go back to work since he was sick so much (it seemed almost 50%) of the fall and winter. When sick, he needed a good deal of attention: to keep him calm (some medicines made him awfully shakey), to force fluids, tempt his appetite, keep track of progress and medicines, scratch and rub his back (gets quite itchy), keep him relatively happy (not being able to play with friends is sad), and in general to soothe, comfort, nurse and get him well.

All this attention and special food and drink, drove his sister into fits of jealousy. The sicker he was, and the more attention he required, the more concern I showed, and the more attention she demanded, or tried to demand. To illustrate this: we left the children with my mother for a few days. He got sick, which my mother was quite competent to handle. She comforted and treated and in general was nurse for the day. She finally had him settled and quiet in our bed watching television. She got to the dishes, suds up to elbows, and Cassandra appears with "let's bake," Mother naturally replied "not now, dear." After some wheedling, healthy sister goes and cons the sick one out of bed. Mother turns around to see Michael snaking on his stomach, head on pillow, wheezing away, going to play with sister dear. When I spoke to my mother, she said she could handle Michael; but Cassie, the one she always thought sweet and close to perfect, was driving her mad.

Michael also has numerous food allergies which require his having different (sister considers them special, better) meals occasionally. Maybe they could be considered special because if you're making a substitute meal for someone, it's silly to make something they don't like. Well, if you cook special for one, why won't you cook special for two. Why does she have to eat things she doesn't particularly like when he doesn't. No amount of talk will convince her that he can't eat it, it will make him sick, but it's good for her. So, you cook special for her too sometimes.

Another difference I noted with Michael is that he wasn't invited for dinner or overnight as often as a well child (this seemed to straighten out as he got older). Other mothers were nervous; they won't know what to feed him or what to do if he gets sick.

I tried to make it clear that he's just a little boy who is sometimes sick. Not a sickly child. He wanted to do, and could do, the same things as other little boys. He was just as strong and healthy (when not wheezing) as anyone else. Kids with asthma have a bad image.

Asthma is not cheap with specialists, allergy shots, preventatives, emergency visits, check-ups, medicines for attacks. This also has some effect on the family. Some of your priorities have to be down-shifted to slip these expenses up on the list.

So, time, keeping child and siblings happy and healthy and cost are probably, in that order, the main effects of having asthma in our family.

On the positive side, as he's gotten older a good preventative treatment program has been established. I've become aware of the do's and don'ts and he has also. He's aware of the early signals and is able to initiate early treatment. He is less often ill, requires less time and less special treatment. This eases some of the jealousy. He's happier because he's not missing out on things. His asthma is not important to his peers. It doesn't effect his performance in school or sports. He's accepted for himself.

JOSEPH

by Gail Platz

My son Joseph is five years old and has had occasional asthma attacks since he was one and a half. In August he had a mild attack and as usual it woke us up at 3 a.m. My first response was, maybe it's just croup again, so we steamed up the bathroom for 15 minutes and tried to read through the fog. Unfortunately that didn't stop the cough or slow his breathing rate down to normal, but he did manage to get back to sleep for a while. I have in my medicine chest an array of medicines but I wasn't sure which one to use or how much. Since it was still the middle of the night I didn't want to wake the doctor whom I had just met the week before. At last Joey went back to sleep. The following day we took him in to see the doctor, got his medicine straightened out and his asthma under control.

In October we attended the parents' asthma group. Finally, we were learning what was going on and how to deal with it effectively. One of the worst things about the asthma had always been not understanding it. We learned also about the various medications which are used, how to use them, and perhaps most important, what their effects are. Joey, we discovered, hadn't been at an effective dose level and his symptoms would hang on and on. We got a 'practice' inhaler and he has now mastered the technique for getting medicine directly into his lungs. We also have a home huffer which he can now use correctly although it took a while to learn.

Perhaps the most valuable part of the parents' asthma group was finally getting to ask all those questions which arise but you don't feel there is time for in an office visit, or they get forgotten until the next episode. I learned a lot from other people's experiences and how they handled their situations. Another important element was involving both parents. This helped me to share the responsibility I had felt was primarily mine.

In November Joey had a moderate asthma attack which my husband was first to notice. This time around everything was easier to deal with since we had a better understanding of what was going on with our son. We were able to bring the attack under control fairly quickly, and with much less anxiety. Joey was soon off to bed and slept peacefully all night.

MICHAEL
By Sherry Polito

My son, Michael was two years old when he had his first asthma attack. During that time, he had a bad cold. I heard some wheezing while he was breathing, and made an appointment to see the doctor. The wheezing got progressively worse and he was having more difficulty breathing. I tried to keep him and myself calm. Finally, after receiving three shots of epinephrine, Michael's wheezing subsided. I thought to myself, I don't want Michael to go through this nightmare again. The doctor told me that he definitely had an asthma attack. I shuddered, thinking what that poor little boy was in for and how my husband and I could cope with this.

My husband and I are both registered nurses. I worked in a hospital atmosphere for many years and had taken care of many patients with asthma. With all this experience I was still scared when I heard that Michael had asthma.

Asthma runs on both sides of our family. My husband's sister was very sick with it. My husband remembered how his parents would take her from one doctor to another trying to give her some relief. To this day, his sister is still under treatment. I saw what my parents went through with my brother. He was always so pale and thin and was constantly catching colds. He missed a lot of school due to his asthma. At times he was quite unmanageable. My mother gave into a lot of his whims, fearing that he would bring on an asthma attack if she was firm.

With all this in mind I didn't want to accept the fact that Michael had asthma. I felt guilty for not bringing him to the doctor's sooner and for thinking the way I did. I felt very nervous wondering how I was going to handle his next attack.

My pediatrician recommended that my husband and I attend an asthma workshop that he was giving. Even when I started the classes I still didn't think that Michael had asthma. The asthma workshop was quite helpful to us. We were able to share our feelings and listened to others with similar problems and some with more severe problems. The discussion group helped us understand more about asthma and helped us learn when to give the medication Michael needed

I didn't want to start medication so late that it wouldn't be effective and I didn't want to give it every time he had a stuffy nose. I was afraid he would have too much theophylline in his system. After the workshop was over I had a clearer perspective as to how I was going to handle Michael. I was able to cope with my son's episodes of asthma better. My husband

and I both decided that to prevent an attack from getting worse we should treat earlier.

From Michael's asthma records, it seems that Michael goes into his asthma attacks after he catches a cold. Allergies do not effect him so far. We try to prevent his asthma from getting worse by giving him his medication when he starts showing cold symptoms. This has worked for us. We try not to treat Michael any different from his brother. When Michael is on the medication we let his nursery school teachers know, for he tends to be very high strung and very active. He is treated just like all the other children and we have had no problems with Michael in nursery school.

We are pleased at the present time with how we are handling Michael's illness. He seems to be doing better now that he is four and his trips to the doctor are less frequent.

CHRISTY

By Cecelia Cobbs

Christy is almost four years old. She was born two months prematurely, weighing two pounds, eleven ounces at birth.

She came home from the hospital two months later. She wasn't breathing normally when she came home. Her lungs were under-developed at birth and it was felt that time would strengthen her lungs and the breathing would straighten itself out.

Christy seemed to catch colds easily and with them came the difficulty in breathing (increasing difficulty at night). It was very scary for both of us. The harder it was to breathe the more upset Christy would get and the breathing would become even more difficult. We spent many a night in a rocking chair.

She was about six months old when asthma was mentioned. I had mixed feelings about asthma. Relief in knowing what the problem was but also very worried as I knew nothing about it, nor did I know anyone else who had it.

Christy experienced very undesirable side effects from the first couple of drugs she was given. This was very frightening and frustrating. After trying several different drugs we found one that Christy could tolerate.

It seemed every time she got a cold, the asthma would surface. When Christy was about two years old she had a prolonged bout with a cold and asthma. She ended up in the hospital with pneumonia. I was very scared, I think more than Christy. She didn't want to stay in the hospital, but we stayed together which was good for both of us.

Around this time I went to the asthma classes at the Amherst Medical Associates. This helped me a great deal, which ultimately helped Christy. I felt much more relaxed and understood much more about it. And it's comforting being around other people who understand and deal with the same feelings.

Since attending the sessions I've found I don't think about Christy having asthma until it surfaces. Before I think it was always on my mind and I was constantly waiting for it to happen.

The asthma has subsided in the past year. Christy has had fewer colds and hasn't been bothered nearly as much with asthma. And at this point I am very optimistic.

BABYSITTERS AND OTHERS

As you know, most neighbors, babysitters and relatives have little knowledge of asthma. What do they need to know about asthma in order to interact properly with your child? The amount of information you give will depend on the severity and frequency of attacks, time spent in their care, and availability of people who can help in case of a problem.

A babysitter should have some general knowledge about asthma as outlined in "What is Asthma" (see Chapter 2). S/He should also have specific information about medications: time and method of administration; desired effects and side effects. Instructions about whom to call in case of an asthma attack. Adequate instruction for a babysitter or overnight visit can be supplied by filling in the form below.

Neighbors and children who are in contact with but not responsible for your child should understand that asthma usually does not interfere with normal activity. Interested adults should have the opportunity to read, "What is Asthma," and discuss your child's status with you.

INSTRUCTIONS FOR OVERNIGHT OR BABYSITTER

_____ has _____asthma.

S/He takes the following medicines on a regular basis:

Theophylline, as _____ ____ mg. at _____ and _____.

Adrenergic inhaler, as _____ a double whiff every four hours with an attack.

If _____ has difficulty breathing:

- makes a noise breathing out
- sucks in the skin above the collarbone
- takes longer to breathe out than breathe in

Please call me for instructions at _____. If you can not reach me, call Dr. _____ at _____.

Please see attached sheets for more information on asthma, medications, and when to give them.

Chapter Five
AWAY FROM HOME - INTRODUCTION

Parents need a plan to deal with asthma attacks which occur while their child is away from home. Written instructions are more important in this situation than when you are in familiar surroundings.

Emily's Thanksgiving visit would have gone more smoothly if her mom had been carrying a letter describing the usual treatment for her asthma attack. Review of this bad experience helped us prepare for the next visit. It went fine. Monica's mom was apprehensive about sending her off to California with newly diagnosed asthma. She outlines her preparations.

Asthma attacks do occur in school. The school staff needs explicit instructions if they are to respond appropriately. Monica kept her asthma a secret and had problems with an attack. After good communication between her mom and the principal, Monica will be able to handle future attacks effectively. Sample instructions for a school nurse are presented.

Teachers should know about asthma in order to react properly to their students' complaints. An Information for Teacher sheet outlines the situation. Often a child with asthma can give a report to teach his class about this common problem. In the process he will learn more about his asthma and may become better able to control it. David's report is an example.

EMILY

The Thanksgiving Disaster

by Gail Hall

The decision to visit my brother in New York for the Thanksgiving holiday was in some ways a difficult one and in some ways easy. I remembered our last visit to New York when six-year-old Emily had an asthma reaction to my brother's cats. This was not terribly pleasant since we ended up in the emergency room instead of at the table for Easter dinner. Based on that experience, I knew trouble was a real possibility, but it was definitely time to get out of town. Visiting my brother, his wife and their new baby was a treat, too, since the rest of my family is in the Chicago area, a two-day drive from our Western Massachusetts university town.

Part of the experience of travelling had always been that I knew that a situation might be borderline when no one else did. Even though my brother and sister-in-law had worked with me for some time to make the presence of their two elegant cats and new puppy as small a problem as possible, I still felt it was my responsibility to manage each subtle health situation without letting it dominate everyone's experience of the visit. I found it difficult to say, "Oh, excuse me, let me just listen to her breathing here," or, "I wonder where she is in the house." I imagined myself walking in the door saying, "Hi! So glad to see you. Could you get that rug out of here? Is your humidifier working?"

I planned for trouble as best I could. I let my brother know I wouldn't make the final decision about coming until the last minute. If Emily developed a cold we would have to cancel since I knew a cold would send her over the edge if she were with cats. I also put her on the metaproterenol inhaler for three days before we were scheduled to leave. I moved her dose up gradually, from one day to the next, until she was using it three times a day, two whiffs each time. This gradual approach helps prevent side effects. I decided to use the inhaler even though I knew it meant a better than 50% chance of getting up two or three times during the night because she doesn't sleep well when she's taking the inhaler. That was just part of the deal. I also let my brother know it was likely to be a very brief trip.

We took the bus to New York and arrived Thanksgiving midday. After lunch it was time for her second dose of the inhaler. We had been in the house only about an hour, but the inhaler let me know that things were already happening. After she takes a whiff, Emily tries to hold her breath for ten seconds and I count. After the first whiff, she had some trouble holding her breath as long as usual, but after the second whiff, things had improved. This change let me know that her breathing was being affected by the environment.

So I knew we were having some difficulty. I could have tuned into the situation more clearly at that point and said it was time to leave, but I really didn't want to. I told myself that perhaps I had miscounted or perhaps the inhaler would see us through, along with the theophylline which she took every day. My brother and sister-in-law were pleased to announce the arrival of their new humidifier which they had positioned in the guest room. The cats had been kept out of the guest room since the previous summer. And my sister-in-law had even washed the guest room walls that morning. It was definitely not time to go home.

The rest of the day was the kind of balancing act I had feared it would be. When I took the suitcases upstairs to the guest room, the room was indeed moist and clean, right down to the tenacious cat hairs which my all too wary eye detected. I kept an eye on Emily, shooed her away from the cats and tried to limit her time with the dog she adored. After a while I sent her upstairs to the guest room to watch TV. After our Thanksgiving dinner, the second use of the inhaler told me things were a little worse. When asked, Emily said she was fine: as far as Emily is concerned, what is ignored will go away. I began to think of ways to stay out of the house the next day.

In the morning, Emily was having so much trouble breathing that even my sister-in-law knew she was fibbing when Emily said she was fine. As we worked on the second round of the Thanksgiving dishes, we devised a plan for getting everybody out of the house and on the road, in hopes of giving Emily's breathing a chance to get back to normal. The weather was nice enough to go to the Bronx Zoo, so we got people fed and left for the day. We'd be outside, and everyone, including Emily's eleven-year-old sister, Adrianne, could have a good time. I was being a little too optimistic, however. The event could have been entitled, "The Salvation Army Goes to the Zoo." Emily was having so much trouble breathing that she had trouble walking up the hills the zoo provided. My brother carried her while Adrianne limped along behind in the leg brace she was wearing for her troublesome but not serious knee problem, chondromalacia of the patella. I watched the clock, deciding whether to leave enough time for a trip to my sister's pediatrician if things didn't improve. But we were having too good a time and I figured the worst that could happen if we stayed was an evening trip to the emergency room as we had done last Easter. On that trip she received a shot of Susphrine, a long-acting form of epinephrine that got us through the night. So we stayed at the zoo and I was glad to see Adrianne having a good time while we forgot as best we could about asthma for a while.

At five o'clock, everyone was tired. We used the inhaler again but things weren't getting better. In fact, they were worse. The inhaler ceased being useful because Emily could no longer hold her breath long enough to let the medication stay in the bronchial tubes and have its effect. In a last effort to play for time, I suggested we go for ice cream. Well of course, any fool who decides to stop and get something to eat in New York gets what she deserves. There were no ice cream parlors anywhere. My brother doesn't know ice cream parlors; his kid is only four months old. Emily was getting exhausted and Adrianne was beginning to show signs of wear and tear. She had realized that things had turned and we were now doing asthma. So every time we got in and out of the car looking for an ice cream, she followed Emily into the back seat with, "You little jerk, you're faking it." The third time she did I offered to punch her in the mouth. Things had deteriorated.

Finally, we found a delicatessen. Emily, now without an appetite, managed to eat some jello and Adrianne enjoyed some New York cheesecake. I let my brother know that things were definitely not okay and we left for home, not really sure what to do. We arrived at home but a half hour later my brother drove Emily and me to the hospital, with Emily lying in the backseat, gasping short breaths, no longer pretending she was okay.

We drove to the hospital in Bronxville where we had been at Easter. The same doctor, of course, who was there in April was not there now and things looked pretty busy in the emergency room. I brought Emily in and after the usual insurance procedures I told the nurse that Emily was having trouble with asthma, that I thought she needed an injection, that we had been there before, that she took theophylline a 200 mg. tablet twice a day and that she used a metaproterenol inhaler, but it was no longer useful to us because she was unable to hold her breath.

The nurse spoke with the intern or resident and he came over and asked me what I thought the problem was. I repeated what I had said to the nurse and added that I felt that, given Emily's previous experience with asthma, the situation warranted an injection of adrenalin. "I think she needs a shot because the oral medication we've been using is no longer working," I said. "I think you need to calm down," was his response.

I had entered the emergency room aware that I had to play a low key role because I knew some physicians found it difficult to deal with parents who have a lot of information, and, God help them, an opinion. I understood that it was important to avoid acting as if I were going to be the one to make a decision. Instead, it was my role to simply feed information, and very slowly at that. I understood it was important not to irritate the people who had the drug my kid needed. In retrospect, I see that I should have followed this insight more closely and not suggested the shot. At any rate, I was not prepared for the level of hostility that I met, partly because it was not there on my last visit, and partly because I'm never prepared for hostility.

We had to wait another fifteen minutes for the physician who was on duty. He was moving from bed to bed and it seemed that he had spoken with the nurse and the intern or resident. The fact that it was hard to tell who was who or who had talked with whom illustrates a device that I think people either consciously or subconsciously use in emergency rooms, that is, that no one identifies themselves in terms of rank or name. They simply move at you and away from you without letting you know what the plan is, who they are, who is making decisions, or what's going on. He finally came over and listened very briefly to Emily's chest. His diagnosis was, "This isn't an asthma attack." As he walked away with an air of disdain, he remarked over his shoulder, "She's hyperventilating."

I was amazed that he did not notice her retractions or that her inhale/exhale ratio was reversed, two signs of real trouble breathing. They occur with asthma but not with hyperventilation. I knew why he said she wasn't having an asthma attack. It was because she wasn't wheezing. But wheezing isn't necessary to an asthma attack; in fact, you can only wheeze if some air goes through the windpipes. Emily wasn't wheezing because many of her windpipes were completely closed.

I started to say something but he was gone. I was trying to hold out for a rational explanation for what was going on, but it was difficult. Perhaps the emergency room was truly overloaded with emergencies, however all I noted were two discussions of how to apply ace bandages and where to go for a throat culture. While the physician was gone, the nurse gave Emily oxygen through a nasal device. He returned, after another fifteen minutes, and took the device off Emily, saying, "We don't need this." He started firing questions at me about her medications and interrupting me every time I tried to answer. Finally he said, "We'll give her an injection. We can x-ray her, too." After more delays and confusion she got the injection and x-ray. To no one's surprise, she did not have pneumonia - and we left. I thought that even though it had been a truly unpleasant experience, it was over. I figured that we were home free. She would sleep through the night as she had done at Easter and we would leave right away in the morning.

We went back to my brother's house and I put Emily to bed. Soon thereafter, I went to sleep in the room with her. What I thought would be a night of much-needed sleep turned into a nightmare. Emily woke at midnight in real distress, and beginning to panic. She was struggling to catch her breath with little success. The inhale/exhale ratio was reversed. She was exhaling with such difficulty that it was as if somebody was punching her in the stomach every time she tried to exhale. I was becoming upset because I couldn't help her and things weren't making any sense. Plus I was going to have to get my brother out of bed and go back out in the cold.

When we got back to the emergency room the intern, I could see, was not pleased to see us but somewhat softened in his response. The other physician was gone for the night. The nurses were solicitious as usual and trying to be useful. I came with the fear that the intern would decide that the next step would be to give Emily more injected medication. On several occasions when she had had more than one shot in one day she had developed severe side effects. While most kids get cranky and nervous, Emily gets paranoid. She imagines that she is in danger, that everything around her is rotting. Her legs shake. She has fits of anger. It usually starts with a headache, pain in her chest and vomitting, and lasts for an hour or more. In short, a bad drug trip. I had gotten used to the vomitting - vomitting on the sidewalk is part of living with asthma - but I had never gotten used to the terror.

I went in to the emergency room thinking about how I would have to deal with people who really didn't want to see me again. Last time, I just had to wait it out until they gave her the medicine. This time I was going to have to try to change their minds. I wanted them to admit her to the hospital, and give her medication intravenously. When she had been hospitalized in October, IV medication had brought the breathing under control and there had been no side effects. Also, if she were in the hospital she would be away from the cats, which were the source of the problem. I knew I couldn't go back to my brother's house.

I presented my case to the intern: "I don't think she should have another injection. I know from my experience with injections that it might cut the symptoms in half at best, and, I don't know for sure, but she may have severe side effects which, given the situation, how uncomfortable she is now, seems really like a bad idea." "Well, who's the doctor here?" shouted the resident or intern or whoever he was. I said, "I can tell you from my experience that we're not going to have any success with just injections. I can't go home. I either have to go to a motel room in the middle of the night or she has to spend the night in the hospital." Well," he said, "we'll have to call in the pediatrician who is on call." I felt bad, I don't know why, about getting somebody else out of bed on a cold night.

The pediatrician came in about a half an hour later and said, "Have you had this child desensitized?" It is 1:00 a.m. and a lecture on how he thought asthma should be dealt with was not of interest to me. I wanted my kid relieved of her distress. He ordered an injection, she got it and we waited to see if she would respond. I hadn't fought it anymore since I didn't see any other way to make progress and she needed something to help her breathe right away. The pediatrician was reluctant to hospitalize her. "I can't just hospitalize someone; she would have to stay for the whole day. We would have to do a lot of blood tests." What he really meant was he couldn't hospitalize her just because her mother wanted it. After her second injection, Emily was much better. I leaned down to hug her and said, "You're being a real trooper." "That's enough compliments for now," she said, ever articulate. The decision was made not to hospitalize her so my brother and I headed for the Yonkers Holiday Inn. Miraculously, the side effects never occured.

The doctors, for all their obnoxious attitudes, had followed standard protocol for the treatment of asthma. As far as they were concerned, I was a crazy woman off the street, hysterical with a hysterical child. I don't know that I would have had much more luck in dealing with anyone, my sister-in-law's pediatrician or anybody else. It's difficult to talk anyone into skipping standard protocol for the treatment of asthma, and that's the dilemma of being away from home. As we arrived at the Holiday Inn, I seriously considered giving up travelling forever.

My brother left us and Emily and I quickly went to sleep. But at 4:30 she woke again and this time in severe distress and panicky. At this point, the difference between hyperventilation, panic and asthma doesn't matter. I spent a half an hour trying to get her to breath calmly, but again the inhale/exhale ratio was reversed and her breathing was shallow, rapid and out of control. The interval gave me time to think. I considered going to Montefiore Hospital which Emily's pediatrician had suggested in case of emergency. Now I was sorry I hadn't followed his advice. But the fact was I had gotten her away from the cats, the injections were now part of a pattern lasting four hours and she wasn't having side-effects.

The IV would have solved all this but it was too late for that now. I might as well go back and get another injection. I called my sister-in-law just to touch base with the world of the sane and then called the cab company. We arrived in a taxi at 5:30 a.m. The nurse who had been there the whole time stared at us sadly as we came in. Emily went to the bed she had been on before. Her tears fell on the floor as she told the nurse that she could never go back to her uncle's house to play with the dog. The intern looked sympathetic. I wasn't angry or interested in proving that I had been right. At this point I felt as if I were sleepwalking, going through the motions I had gone through before. She got the shot and they didn't record it. We were not billed for that visit but the other two visits came to $156.00. The motel room was $62.00.

I had asked the taxi to wait outside. She vomitted on the side walk and we got back in the cab for another $5.00 ride across Yonkers as the sun began to rise over New York. Emily said, "This is a big cab, Mom." I said, "Yeah, well, you probably wouldn't get to ride in a big yellow cab with jump seats unless we were doing this, so let's think of it that way." Back at the Holiday Inn I called my brother to let him know we were back and I called the bus station to find out when we could get a bus. So far I'd had three hours of sleep. I was on automatic pilot. I'm glad my kid hadn't vomitted in the backseat of the cab, I thought to myself, but frankly, I didn't care.

I fell asleep and slept a couple of hours. At 10:30 I called my brother and said, "Things are better but we'll have to move fast to catch the 12:30 bus." My brother picked us up and we drove to his house. Emily waited in the car while I ran in and threw everything in suitcases. My sister-in-law, as always, had the turkey sandwiches and celery sticks and ginger ale packed for us and my brother took a picture of Emily with her beloved friend, Peaches, the golden retriever. We all piled into the car and headed for the George Washington Bridge Bus Terminal. When we got there, found a parking space and the ticket window, they said, "Sorry, that bus is filled. That's the express bus, you know."

Through all this Adrianne had been a real saint. She spent the morning helping my sister-in-law with the baby and getting things organized. I hadn't seen her for 12 hours; she basically got crossed out of the picture. While we waited for the bus, I tried to spend some time talking to her with one eye on Emily. My brother and I discussed what should happen if Emily had trouble on the way home. If things got real bad on the bus, I could ask the bus driver to take me to the police and they would get me to a hospital. At this point I didn't care who got inconvenienced. The whole world could stop while I got the treatment I needed for my kid.

The bus ride back was not bad: five hours on the local route, eating turkey sandwiches. I got as many cans of soda as I could into Emily to keep her from getting dehydrated; she actually ate some bits of turkey, to my surprise. We got back and it was 7 p.m. before everyone was settled at home. I managed to get a little more food into Emily before the post-asthma-attack complaining session began. She had behaved like a soldier through the worst of it, but safe at home she began to whine and cling. There is a closeness between mother and child in a severe illness that's like infancy: so much attention must be paid to the child's body, long periods of time are spent in close quarters. Then suddenly it's over. Emily wasn't sure she was ready. I was totally exhausted, Adrianne was edgy, and Emily wanted to sit on my lap. But this was part of the deal. Somehow we got through the evening and Emily went to bed and slept well.

The next day it was hard to tell she had had asthma. Allergic reactions come and go quickly. I sent her to a babysitter's and went to work. But Monday night she had a bad time trying to sleep, apparently a delayed reaction to the whole event. Three or four nightmares, restless sleeping, waking up and talking in her sleep. But that was the end of it, at least for her. I needed about a week of sleep.

Could any of it been changed? When I talked with Emily's pediatrician, he was disappointed that I hadn't called him from the hospital. I had indeed thought about it but it seemed like a crazy idea. He couldn't drive to Yonkers and I couldn't imagine how it would have made things better to have him talk to the doctors on the phone to tell them how to do their jobs. But in thinking about it more, I realized that he could have talked to them and they might indeed have listened. He could have given them a sense of her history and they might have at least have been able to treat her more effectively. Doctors talk to doctors when they don't talk to civilians--that's the way it is.

I had written a few "Dear Doctor" letters for my patients before the Thanksgiving disaster. Emily's experience provoked me to make it a more regular habit. I am willing to write this letter for any child whose parent has taken the Asthma Course. My secretary types it up after I fill in the blanks. The form and Emily's completed letter are on the following pages.

The best way to deal with an emergency room is to stay away from it. Emergency rooms often do an excellent job of taking care of very sick people. They do not do as well in caring for patients who are moderately ill. One often has to wait a long time for service because people with critical injuries or illness are taken first (as they should be). Follow-up arrangements and advice are often inadequate. If you know how to take care of your child's asthma, you may never have to use an emergency room.

If your child does require emergency care by someone other than your usual physician, you should be able to give him/her detailed information so that the care for your child can be individualized. A copy of the Asthma Record and the Emergency Room Doctor letter will provide this necessary information. Emily went back to New York for Thanksgiving in 1982. We did everything we could to prepare for the visit. She and her family stayed at a friend's house, rather than living with her uncle's family and the cat. Before her visit she started using her metaproterenol inhaler every four hours. She started taking cromolyn and prednisone one day before the visit began. The three-day visit was peaceful; Emily didn't wheeze once.

FORM FOR LETTER

Dear Dr.

_____ has _____ asthma.

___ His/Her mother/father has taken a four-hour course on asthma for parents. S/He has a good understanding of the pathophysiology and management of his/her child's asthma.

___ It is controlled by theophylline taken as _____ ___ mg every ___ hours. This amounts to ___ mg/kg/day.

___ His/Her last theophylline level on this dose was ___ on ___.

___ S/He uses a beta-adrenergic inhaler, up to 4 double whiffs a day.

___ S/He takes cromolyn by (nebulizer, Spinhaler) ___ times a day.

___ S/He has received prednisone on ___ occasion in the past year.

___ Early introduction of prednisone in a dose of ___ mg/day has truncated his/her attacks. I usually prescribe for three days.

___ His/Her last peak flow was _____ liters/minute on _____.

___ His/Her attacks come on quickly and s/he sometimes breathes too fast to use the inhaler.

___ S/He has benefitted from metaproterenol/albuterol by nebulizer.

___ His/Her usual dose is ___ cc of a 5% solution in ___ cc of saline, given every 30 minutes, up to 3 times.

___ If s/he benefits from adrenalin given subcutaneously, ___ cc every 15 minutes, up to 3 times, this may be followed by Sus-phrine ___ cc

If you have any questions, please call me or my associates at (413) 253-XXXX at any hour of the day or night. Our office is open six days a week and five nights a week; the answering service can reach us at other times. Please make it clear to the answering service that you are a physician and wish to speak with one of the pediatricians.

Sincerely,

_____, M.D.

LETTER FOR EMILY

June 14, 1984

Dear Doctor:

Emily Hall has had chronic asthma of moderate severity since 1979. In October 1981, she was hospitalized for treatment of status asthmaticus. Her mother has taken a 4-hour course on asthma for parents. She has a good understanding of the pathophysiology and management of her child's asthma and is a contributing author to CHILDREN WITH ASTHMA: A MANUAL FOR PARENTS.

Emily takes cromolyn sodium four times a day. She uses an albuterol inhaler, up to 6 double whiffs a day. Emily takes Theodur 150 mg. every 12 hours (10 mg/kg/day). She has received short bursts of prednisone on four occasions in the past 12 months. Early introduction of prednisone, 40 mg/day, has truncated her attacks.

She measures her peak flow rate at home, morning and night. Normal peak flow is 325 liters/minute with a mini-Wright Peak Flow Meter. A drop of greater than 30% in her peak flow, which does not return to normal following use of the metaproterenol inhaler, indicates that she will develop an attack within the next 24 hours.

Her attacks come on quickly and she sometimes breathes too fast to use the inhaler. In this situation, she may benefit from metaproterenol by nebulizer 0.2 cc in 2.5 cc saline. This can be given three times at 1/2-hour intervals. She has gotten overactive, angry and scared following adrenalin but may benefit from 0.15cc. She does benefit from adrenalin 0.15 cc given twice, 15 minutes apart. If her wheezing clears this may be followed by Susphrine 0.08 cc.

If you have any questions, please call me or one of my pediatric associates at (413) 253-XXXX at any hour of the day or night. Our office is open six days a week and five nights a week; the answering service can reach us at other times. Please make it clear to the answering service that you are a physician and wish to speak with one of the pediatricians.

Sincerely,

Thomas F. Plaut, M.D.

MONICA

The California Trip

By Celine Cyran

The winter of 1981-1982 thirteen-year-old Monica was diagnosed as having asthma. I first panicked and thought, not that too. One and a half years ago, she was diagnosed with scoliosis. I thought isn't that bad enough? Now that we have that under control, why this? I just remembered my brother when he was young and the attacks he had.

Monica was planning on spending the summer in California with my sister, Marielle. I wondered if this would change her plans. She was looking forward to the trip for a long time, but how could I send her 3,000 miles away for someone else to take care of her when I didn't understand what was happening to her myself.

We weathered her first attack with the pediatrician's guidance and reassurance that asthma can be controlled. I started reading all the material he recommended and slowly began understanding what was happening to Monica.

A few months later, Monica had another attack. Naturally my first reaction was to panic again, but I called the doctor and we again got through this one all right. In the meantime, my sister was trying to confirm all the plans for Monica to fly out to California. I still didn't feel comfortable with all of this. I really knew I needed to learn more so I could cope with Monica's trip.

Our pediatrician had scheduled a four-hour course for parents of children who have asthma. The sessions that were held by him and his partner were very productive. It was reassuring to hear concerns and share feelings with other parents.

They recommended using a stethoscope to learn how to pick up problems with breathing early. Then medication could be given in the beginning stages. Also the huffer was recommended to measure the breathing (peak flow), to help make decisions on medications. Right away my thoughts were on Monica's trip to California. If I bought the huffer, Monica could monitor her own breathing. After all, I thought, she's almost 14 years old. I was starting to feel better.

After a lengthy consultation with the pediatrician reassuring me everything would be fine, Monica left with instructions for herself, my sister, explanation from the doctor about the type of asthma Monica has, explanation of side effects and how to handle it if a problem occurred. She also had necessary phone numbers, a letter from the pediatrician to an emergency room physician, and my permission releasing responsibility to my sister for emergency room treatment. Naturally I felt much better about everything.

By the time Monica boarded the plane, I felt confident that if an attack occurred:

- Monica could start treating herself.
- If Monica didn't panic, my sister wouldn't panic.
- My sister would be reassured that Monica knew how to take care of herself and could always read the material I sent her.
- They had all the necessary forms and information they would need in case of an emergency.
- I had covered all bases.

When Monica handed my sister the information folder, my sister reacted and said, "What's all this?" Monica replied, "You'd do the same if it was your daughter."

Mrs. Cyran's Letter to her sister and general instructions for the care of Monica's asthma appear below:

Marielle,

Thanks for taking Monica for such a long time this summer. This should be quite an experience for her...

I hope I've sent the information you need as far as Monica's asthma is concerned. I hope it doesn't scare you away. With luck, you won't need any of this. I really hope so, it took me a while to understand what was happening.

There are a few environmental factors that will trigger asthma: house dust (can't get away from), mold and <u>cigarette smoke</u>. When, and <u>if</u> she's having difficulty breathing, she should stay away from smoke.

I've enclosed a permission release form for emergency use. (Hope you won't have to use.)

Monica knows how to use her medicine, she should also know when she needs it. If she uses her huffer to monitor her breathing, she'll be all set.

About a week before she comes back, you can check with the airline to reserve a seat for her in the non-smoking section. Also, she likes window seats.

Enough instructions. Have a good summer.

Lots of Love,

Celine

GENERAL INSTRUCTIONS FOR TREATING
AN ASTHMA ATTACK

Monica is being treated for asthma. It is of mild severity.

An attack usually comes on after exercise or with an infection.

When she starts to wheeze, she should take Theodur one half of a 300 mg. tablet every 12 hours. It should be continued for 1 day after the wheezing stops.

She should use the inhaler one double whiff every fours hours while awake for the first day and then up to four times a day if still wheezing.

If she is not greatly improved after 24 hours of treatment, please contact Dr. Plaut, or Dr. Jones at 413-253-XXXX.

While taking medication for an asthma attack, she should drink at least 64 ounces of liquid a day.

The Alupent inhaler should be used 15 minutes before strenuous exercise to prevent wheezing. The effect usually lasts four hours.

Please check the handouts for side effects of medication.

Call me if you have any questions.

Our schools are trying to do a good job of educating our children. Obviously, absences interfere with a student's learning. Sporadic absences are particularly disruptive. We try to keep children in school as much as possible. This means that they return during an asthma attack and do not miss for minor episodes.

To keep an asthma attack under control, the student often has to take medication during the school day. In addition, her activity may have to be temporarily reduced.

What is a proper medication policy for a school? I believe that all junior and senior high school students should be able to carry and regulate their own medication. It is too cumbersome and embarassing for them to check in with the school nurse for each dose of medicine. However, a record of all drugs a student is taking should be on file in the health office.

In general, elementary school students should go to the nurse's room for medication. This will cut down on abuse of the inhaler, and also insure that the medication is taken at the proper time. Those students who are responsible enough to take their medicine as directed should be allowed to do so. This may be negotiated between parent, school nurse and doctor.

I try to arrange medication schedules so that a minumum of medication is taken during school hours. Theophylline usually can be taken every twelve hours. The inhaler is used every four hours during an attack. If it is used before school it should only be used once during the school day. It should be available to prevent exercise-induced asthma. Cromolyn and prednisone may be used twice during the school day.

The biggest problem teachers have is to know when

- a student should be kept inside
- a student should be excused from gym
- a student should be sent to the nurse's room
- a parent should be notified of the problem.

The school staff cannot make these judgments without guidance from the student's parent. Each of these situations can be anticipated. If the school staff receives explicit instructions they perform very well. For an example of one school's response to a problem, see the account of Monica's episode and the subsequent correspondence between her mom and the principal.

The school health staff in the Amherst school system raised the following questions during an inservice program:

How do you relieve anxiety in a child who is having an attack?

- The school nurse must have a written plan of action supplied by the parent for taking care of an asthma attack. It should include quiet talk, administration of warm liquids, administration of medications as prescribed and contact with the parent if there is no improvement.

How do you deal with gym teachers who don't believe that a child is having trouble, or alternatively, restrict the child's activities when it doesn't seem to be necessary?

- Gym teachers spend a lot of time dealing with students who prefer rest to exercise. Ideally, the parent and doctor will have defined, in writing, the situations in which the student should be excused. Most children with asthma can participate in gym except in the middle of an attack. Children with exercise-induced asthma should take theophylline or use an inhaler before gym to prevent problems.

What do you do with a medication that is not properly labelled?

- Medications should be labelled with name, strength, amount to be given and the time of administration. Inadequately labelled medication should be returned to the parent for proper labelling.

What are the side effects of the various medications?

- The most troublesome for the school staff is the hyperactivity produced by theophylline in some children. This is often lessened with a twelve-hour dosing interval or by substituting cromolyn for theophylline in the treatment plan.

What can be done about students who start wheezing in cold weather when travelling to school?

- The student can wear a surgeon's mask or a painter's mask. This creates a resevoir of warm air and thus reduces the amount of cold air reaching the bronchioles. Of course, most kids wouldn't be caught dead wearing one of these masks unless it is hidden by a scarf.

It was Friday and ever since second period gym, I was having a hard time breathing, but I was too busy and too embarrassed to go and use my inhaler between classes, because we only have three minutes to run to our lockers and get our books for next period. By the time fifth period English came, I realized I'd better get my inhaler or die on the spot. That's when I went to my teacher, to ask for a pass to my locker. Of course she said no. I've tried to get out of her classes before. She yelled at me and said I should go sit because I had tried to get out and visit my friends during first period lunch (this is normally true, but this time it was different). I asked her a second time if I could go to my locker and get my inhaler. She screamed no again. She was especially grouchy because there were so many people around her desk. By that time, if she didn't let me go, I was gonna go without her permission and worry about it later. Then I thought, she already hates me anyway. I'd better try one more time. So I screamed at her, "I have asthma." (It took just about everything I had to say this.) "I have to get to my inhaler, I'm having an attack." She replied, "Go, go, go ahead!!!! I don't care what you do anyway!!" So I booked.

While running down three flights of stairs to get to the freshman lockers in the basement (they make us start at the bottom), I thought I'd never make it there. I was having a hard time breathing. I know that sounds dramatic, but I felt lousy!

I got there and just really wanted that medicine in my lungs to feel better. I felt so dizzy, the nurse's aide saw me and brought me to her office. She sat me down and I was so weak I fell down and I passed out. All that was because:

1) I do not bother to carry my inhaler - I know I should.
2) I took my medicine carelessly. It's too late now to say what I should have done, but everyone says, you learn valuable lessons from dumb mistakes.

P.S. As I'm thinking this episode out, I realize the seriousness of this. I've just gone through a very scary situation and never want to have any more asthma-related problems. Only I can control my body, and from now on I want to do the best for me because I don't feel my health is worth any mistakes.

LETTER TO MONICA'S PRINCIPAL

Dear Mr. Murray,

On Friday, 10/8/82, Monica had an asthma attack during her English class. She attempted three times to ask her teacher if she may leave and get her inhaler kept in her locker. By the time she did get to her locker, she was weak. It was fortunate she was near the teachers' room when someone noticed she wasn't feeling well. She was assisted into the room, and helped. By this time it was too late for her to make a quick recovery using the inhaler. She had to come home from school.

I would like to know if there is some way possible all of her teachers could be notified that Monica has asthma, and from time to time needs to use her inhaler. I have attached a permission note from her doctor verifying the fact that it's doctor's orders. You'll note it's dated 8/30/82. Monica did not feel the need to bring it in before this incident.

I do realize that it's hard for teachers to be able to comply with students' wishes every time they want to leave the classroom. In being fair in my request, I would also expect to be notified if the teacher felt Monica was abusing this request.

Any help you can offer will be greatly appreciated. If you feel a conference is necessary, please let me know.

Thank you in advance for your cooperation.

Sincerely,

Celine Cyran

October 13, 1982

Mrs. Celine Cyran
186 Shearer Street
Palmer, Massachusetts

Dear Mrs. Cyran:

This letter is relative to your correspondence of October 11, 1982 concerning Monica's asthmatic condition.

Be assured we will make every one of Monica's teachers aware of her chronic condition. On Friday, October 8th, no one in the school was aware of the situation and as a result of it, the same rules and regulations were applied to Monica as to all other students. It wasn't until she made the teacher aware of her condition that she was allowed to leave the classroom.

As of today each of her teachers will be totally aware of her situation.

Sincerely yours,

Alphonse E. Murray, Jr.
Principal

M/b

Comment: Monica is a typical teenager. She did not want the embarrassment of being tagged as having asthma so she didn't give my note to the school nurse. Thus the school had no knowledge of her problem. Second, she has tried to get out of class in the past so her teacher could have difficulty assessing the situation. It sounds like Monica will play it straight in the future. The school administration and staff are now informed of her status and will respond appropriately.

INFORMATION FOR SCHOOL NURSE

Instruction for parents: please use this form as a sample for a letter informing the school nurse what to expect of your child. I suggest that you first fill it out, then copy it over to avoid confusion about things that don't apply.

*   *   *

_____ has (mild, moderate, severe) asthma.

Ordinarily s/he can be as active as any other child and should not have her/his activities restricted in any way.

During an attack, s/he should not go out in the cold or engage in strenous physical activity.

_____ takes the following medicines in school at the times noted:

____ theophylline as _____ mg, at _____.
____ albuterol/metaproterenol by inhaler at _____ and _____.
____ cromolyn by Spinhaler, at _____.
____ prednisone (5 mg) _____ tablets at _____ and _____.
____ S/He uses the inhaler before sports or if s/he is wheezing during physical activity.
____ S/He should _____ carry her/his inhaler all the time, _____ leave it in a locker, _____ keep it in the health room.
____ knows when s/he needs her/his inhaler -- please let her/him use his judgement. S/He is not to use it more than once in a school day unless I have written you a note.

Please let me know if you would like a fuller description of her/his medicines.

I will be glad to give you the handouts which her/his doctor has written and to go over them with you.

In case you have questions, please call me at home _____ or at work _____.

If you can't reach me, please call _____ at _____ who knows what to do.

If that fails, please call her/his doctor, Dr. _____, at _____ for advice.

Sincerely,

_____

INFORMATION FOR TEACHER

Please use this form as a sample for a letter informing the teacher what to expect of your child. I suggest that you fill it out, then copy it over to avoid confusion about things that don't apply.

*   *   *

_____ has (mild, moderate, severe) asthma.

Ordinarily, s/he can be as active as any other child and should not have her/his activities restricted in any way.

During an attack s/he should not engage in strenuous physical activity or play outside in cold weather.

The medicine which s/he takes occasionally causes headaches and stomach aches and can make her/him jumpy.

Please let me know if you consider her/his behavior inappropriate. S/He should not be allowed to misbehave any more than any other kid in the class.

I have left a list of medicines which s/he takes with the school nurse. I would like to discuss _____ asthma with you.

I hope that _____ will be able to give a report on asthma to her/his class. S/He knows a lot about it and we find that her/his friends are interested in hearing how it all works.

Sincerely,

_____

ASTHMA
David Plaut, Age 13

General Facts about Asthma

When someone has asthma, his or her bronchioles are too sensitive. The degree of sensitivity varies from one person to another. Approximately 5% of all children under 15 in the United States have asthma. That means that about 40 of the 800 children in the Amherst Junior High have asthma. Unfortunately, some of them do not even know they have asthma. They may be mistaking their asthma for bronchitis or a bad cough. This may mean that they have to miss activities because they are not taking the right medicine.

When someone is having an asthma attack, three things happen in his/her hyperactive bronchioles. The muscles around the bronchioles get tighter. The cells lining the bronchioles become swollen and they produce more mucus than usual. These three things block air from leaving the lungs. When I have an asthma attack, it feels like the center of my chest is getting squeezed, making me feel every breath I take.

Triggers of Asthma Attacks

Exercise is the most common trigger of asthma. I usually start wheezing when I forget to use my inhaler before a basketball game. Colds can also trigger asthma attacks. Every time I have had a problem with asthma, I had a cold first. Some asthma attacks are triggered by allergens and irritants. Common allergens are grass pollens, tree pollens, animals, feathers and dust. Some common irritants are: pollution, tobacco smoke, paint and gasoline. The actions caused by emotions can cause an attack. The actual emotions have no effect on asthma attacks, so if someone was very mad about something but did not do anything, nothing would happen. But if the person started yelling and crying, that would start an attack. I have experienced this many times when my father told a joke that made me laugh very hard.

Medicines

The four most commonly used medicines for asthma are: theophylline, metaproterenol, prednisone, and cromolyn sodium. All four make it easier for air to pass through the bronchioles.

Theophylline loosens the muscles around the bronchioles. It can be taken orally in liquid, tablet, or capsule form. Theophylline is often the first medication used for continuing asthma. Since the amount of theophylline in the blood can be measured, it is easy to prescribe the exact dosage. Theophylline is usually prescribed to be taken regularly every six to 12 hours. Smoking sometimes doubles the amount of theophylline needed to keep the bronchioles open.

Side effects of the theophylline are: vomitting, loss of appetite, nervousness, lightheadedness, irregular heart beat, upset stomach, stomach cramps, headaches, dizziness, and with an overdose -- convulsions.

Theophylline can take anywhere between thirty minutes and several hours to work. The length of time depends on which form is used.

Metaproterenol also loosens the tightened muscles around the bronchioles. Metaproterenol may be taken in tablet, liquid, or inhalation form.

The inhalation method works differently from the other ways. Instead of getting to the bronchioles through the blood stream, it goes directly down the trachea. This is obviously much faster and has an almost immediate effect. The inhaler can be used as a pre-treatment before exercise.

Side effects of metaproterenol are: shakiness, rapid heartbeat, pounding in chest, nervousness and vomiting.

The liquid and tablet forms take about 30 minutes to work. Their effect lasts from four to six hours. The inhaled form usually lasts four hours.

Prednisone is the only medicine that unswells the cells lining the bronchioles, and decreases the amount of mucous produced. Prednisone also helps other medicines that relax the muscles around the bronchioles. Prednisone has been used for the treatment of asthma for 25 years. It works slowly (six hours) so it is not useful in the beginning of an attack.

Prednisone has almost no side effects when used for a short time (two weeks), but long-term use can have serious effects.

These effects are: slowing of growth, and trouble controlling certain infections. Other, not as serious, side effects are: weight gain, acne, purple stretch marks on the skin, increase in body hair, headaches, mood changes and trouble sleeping.

Cromolyn sodium prevents asthma attacks rather than stopping them after they have started. It is especially helpful for exercise-induced asthma. Cromolyn sodium may be used when daily theophylline is not tolerated well.

Cromolyn sodium is taken orally. A powder-filled capsule is inhaled by using a special inhaler device. It is taken four times a day for continual asthma and used immediately before exercise to prevent exercise-induced asthma.

Side effects of cromolyn sodium are: bad taste, cough, throat irritation, and in some cases, allergic reactions.

Common Misconceptions about Asthma

One very common misconception about asthma is that people with asthma cannot play sports. If medications are used properly, this is not true. On my last year's basketball team, three of the eight players had asthma. In 1972, five Olympic medal winners had asthma.

Another misconception is that there is a good chance of dying from an asthma attack. This is not true. Only some of the bronchioles are effected during an attack, others are still carrying air properly. Only in rare instances has someone died from an asthma attack. Approximately one out of 500,000 children die each year from an asthma attack.

Conclusion

Many people have worse asthma than I do. My asthma is a nuisance, not a serious problem. If you take care of asthma sensibly, you can do anything -- play soccer, basketball or go skiing. But if you forget to take medicine or don't use it right, you can wind up missing things you like.

Chapter Six

ODDS AND ENDS

Common questions about medications, attacks and triggers come up repeatedly. They are answered here. What should you look for in choosing a doctor for your child with asthma? When should you request a consultation with another physician? Who should use a peak flow meter at home? The review of an excellent book about asthma and a glossary complete this chapter.

COMMON QUESTIONS

Medication

Q. When should I start giving medication?

A. Ordinarily you should start treatment according to a set routine as soon as you recognize the first sign of asthma in your child. For some this will be an early clue such as sneezing, coughing, a runny nose. For others it is a sign of asthma itself: wheeze or tight chest.

Q. When should I stop treatment?

A. A general rule is to give medication for at least seven days or until there has been no wheeze for two days. Then skip a dose; if no symptoms recur, you can stop treatment. If symptoms return after a skipped dose; reinstitute treatment until your child is symptom free for two days.

Q. What are the long-term effects of theophylline?

A. Though theophylline has been used for decades, physical effects due to long-term use have not been described.

Q. What is a safe and effective theophylline level in the blood?

A. The therapeutic range is between 10 and 20 micrograms per decaliter. At a serum concentration of less than 10 it may not be effective, and over 20 it may be toxic.

Q. How often should you clean an inhaler?

A. A hot water rinse each day of use will keep your inhaler clean. A dirty inhaler will not deliver enough medicine. To check your inhaler, puff it into the air and see if the usual amount of spray is coming out.

Q. What is the value of cromolyn?

A. Cromolyn blocks the body's reaction to allergens and exercise on a short-term basis. In addition, it may reduce or eliminate the need for theophylline or steroids on a long-term basis.

Q. When should steroids be used?

A. Patients taking full doses of theophylline and beta-adrenergic agents who continue to have symptoms will benefit from steroid use.

Q. What are the side effects of steroids?

A. There are no significant side effects when steroids are used for less than two weeks. For side effects with long-term use, please see the medication chapter.

Q. Why does my child get an attack when he is already taking medication?

A. The dose of medication which controls an attack provoked by one trigger may not be adequate when another trigger is added to the system. Theophylline may control an attack which was triggered by an upper respiratory infection. Additional triggers such as cold air, an allergen or exercise might produce further reaction in the bronchioles which cannot be contained by the original dose of medication.

Q. Is it safe to double the dose of medication?

A. Any medication changes should be worked out in advance with your doctor. Ordinarily, doubling a standard dose of medication would lead to trouble.

Q. Under what circumstances should the level of theophylline in the blood be checked?

A. -- child continues to have symptoms on a standard dose
   -- if dose is increased above standard for age
   -- if there are any signs of toxicity
   -- if child takes high doses of theophylline daily
   If asthma is well controlled on standard doses of theophylline, there is no need to check the blood level.

Q. What purpose does taking less than a "therapeutic dose" of medication serve?

A. By this question I suppose you mean usual dose. Some children inactivate theophylline slowly and require considerably less than the usual dose of 20 mg per kilogram per day for good effect.

Q. Is it okay for a parent independently to administer prednisone as needed?

A. Yes, if you have worked out guidelines for administration with your doctor. It is important to have written guidelines and also a written record of actual use. I have worked out "independent" prednisone use with only 2% of my patients. The rest call beforehand.

Attacks

Q. What is an asthma attack?

A. Any episode of asthma that involves worsening of breathing that interrupts on-going activities or requires some procedure, such as resting or taking medicine, to resume normal and comfortable breathing.

Q. How can you predict an asthma attack?

A. Contact with a trigger which has usually set off an attack in the past makes it likely that one will occur again. A drop in peak flow of more than 20% makes it likely that one will have an attack soon.

Q. What is the usual duration of an asthma attack?

A. Attacks triggered by exercise may last only two hours. Some attacks triggered by an upper respiratory infection may last for two weeks. Each individual seems to have his own pattern or set of patterns.

Q. How can you tell if a child has an asthma attack if there is no wheezing, just a bad cough, congestion or a lousy cold?

A. A cold is an upper respiratory infection, caused by a virus which primarily affects the nose, throat and sinuses. Congestion is the stuffiness caused by swelling of the tissues in the nose. Asthma is often triggered by a cold and thus may occur at the same time. Asthma affects the lower respiratory tract. Its symptoms are not cleared by coughing, sneezing or blowing your nose. Our motto is, "If it gets better with asthma medicine, it is probably asthma."

Q. Why does an attack sometimes follow a virus infection and other times not?

A. An attack may be set off by a strong trigger or by a combination of weak triggers. A cold plus some pollution will trigger an attack when either one alone may not.

Triggers

Q. What allergens should I look out for?

A. If you child starts wheezing after contact with an animal (dog, cat or pony) you can be quite sure that s/he is allergic to that animal's dander.

Q. Will wood heat trigger asthma?

A. If the stove is tight, wood heat causes no more pollution than other types of heat.

Q. How hard should I work to keep my child away from things which trigger his/her asthma attacks?

A. Your caution should match the seriousness of his/her problem. If he gets a severe attack when s/he comes in contact with a cat, you should try to avoid cats. If that is impossible, he should be pretreated with a beta-agonist, cromolyn and perhaps prednisone to block an attack. This can be done only on an occasional, not a regular, basis. Children who wheeze with exercise should use their inhaler before they start practicing or competing.

General

Q. What are the chances that my child will die of asthma?

A. Health statistics show that it is extremely rare for a child to die of asthma in this country. About 70 deaths are reported annually in children between the ages of one and 15 years. Put another way, there will be only one death this year for every 25,000 children with asthma. A child with asthma is twice as likely to die in a motor vehicle accident as s/he is to die of asthma.

Q. Is it possible for a person to outgrow asthma and than have it recur ten or twenty years later?

A. Yes, about half of children with asthma outgrow it over a period of twenty years. Some of these will have attacks again later in life.

Q. How do you get teenagers to take medications which cause headache and stomach ache?

A. The teenager will decide whether s/he prefers the side effects to an attack. I assume that if the attack is mild, s/he will prefer that to the medicine. If the attacks are severe, medicine would be the logical choice. Also remember that there are several medications to choose from. If one is unacceptable, another should be tried.

Q. When do you recommend allergy testing?

A. See page 48.

Q. Do you give shots for cat or dog allergies?

A. No, you should stay away from them.

Q. How often are shots recommended?

A. About 5-10% of our patients take allergy shots.

Q. How many years should a person try the shots before deciding whether to continue or stop?

A. Two years.

Q. Should every child with asthma use a peak flow meter at home?

A. No, we have found it most useful for children with severe chronic asthma and for teenagers. About ten percent of our patients have found the peak flow meter useful. The youngest is three years old.

Q. How can I get my daughter to help herself?

A. Two year olds have learned to let their parents know when they aren't feeling well. Three year olds can use an inhaler and peak flow meter if they have adequate coordination and are properly motivated and trained. Some six year olds can judge their symptoms and take their medications without direct supervision. The child who does not cooperate in the treatment of her asthma does not understand her responsibility in the treatment process. She probably feels that she cannot control her asthma and is angry when other people try to do it for her. She should read the book, Teaching Myself About Asthma, and decide with her parents what responsibility she will take on and what part of it is theirs.

Q. How do you get a teenager to take medication properly?

A. In general, the asthma management schedule should be worked out by the doctor and older teenager. His tasks should be clear. He should realize that if he skips his medication or comes in contact with an allergen, he will probably get an attack. After a couple of attacks, most teenagers figure out what they can do to cut down on frequency and severity. If a teenager doesn't want to take medicine, he should not be bugged. Let him get an attack - it's a good learning experience. It's a good idea for young teens to take over most of the responsibility for their asthma also. This is not always possible.

Q. How do you deal with the feeling of being different?

A. People with asthma are different - in one way. They have hyper-reactive airways. Most of the feeling different that I have seen has been inflicted by well-meaning doctors, teachers or parents. Children with asthma can play all sports and take part in all physical activities no matter how strenuous, unless they are in the middle of an attack. Less than 10% of our patients have to watch their activity closely between attacks.

Q. What is the best humidity for the environment of a child with asthma?

A. The mucous membranes of the body function best in clearing pollutants at a humidity of 25-40%.

Q. Can you suggest a diet to control asthma?

A. Any well-balanced diet would be satisfactory.

Q. Should I allow my son to stay at a friend's house if I know it will trigger an attack?

A. The two things we should know before answering are: 1) How bad are the attacks? Certainly a serious attack which causes your son to miss school and to require a doctor's assistance should be avoided. 2) Can the attack be prevented by taking medication before and during the visit? If so, it is reasonable to permit the visit.

Q. When should I come to see the doctor?

A. If you cannot judge how your child is doing during an attack, you should see the doctor. She may tell you that you are doing fine. This is the time to try to judge the severity of an attack. Your doctor should review retractions, wheezing and the distortion of the I:O ratio with you. Don't go just for treatment. Make sure you learn something at every visit.

Q. How can the child learn to take care of herself?

A. Children learn one step at a time. First they have to be able to recognize the earliest sign of asthma. Then they should learn what to do, depending on their age: tell a parent, drink warm liquid, take medicine.

Q. Why does asthma worsen after finishing medication?

A. If an attack worsens after medication is stopped, it means that the changes in the bronchioles have not yet cleared up. We often suggest that parents skip one dose of medication to see if symptoms will recur by the time the next dose is due. If they do, medication is resumed; if they don't, it can be stopped.

Q. If I get rid of the cat and the house dust, will the asthma go away?

A. If your child's asthma is triggered by contact with the cat or when you clean house, you will see some improvement after you eliminate the cat and dust. However, your child still has hyperreactive airways and may get attacks due to other triggers.

Q. Do children take medicine all year long?

A. Some take it every day, some half the time, and others only for a total of a few days or weeks per year.

Q. When will I be able to handle an attack properly?

A. If you can answer all the questions on the Asthma Quiz (Chapter Three) and have kept accurate records of your observations for two or three attacks, you should be able to handle most attacks at home.

Q. Is there any way to prevent asthma attacks permanently?

A. No.

Q. Is it safe for my child to take antihistamines? The packages all say they shouldn't be used by a child with asthma.

A. Most asthma experts see no problem with using antihistamines between or during asthma attacks. Theoretically they might dry up the secretions in the windpipes and make it harder to cough them up, but this has never been proved.

Q. Can my child use a cough syrup during an attack?

A. Generally it is not a good idea since the cough may be a sign that the asthma is not being adequately treated. Also, the child should be able to cough up the mucus which is blocking the windpipes.

Q. Will children who have short attacks always continue in this pattern?

A. Each child has his/her own pattern or set of patterns. One of my patients has severe three-day attacks triggered by a cat and milder two-week attacks triggered by a cold.

Q. What do you do when travelling?

A. Take your instructions, Asthma Record, and Emergency Room Doctor letter with you, as well as an adequate supply of all your child's medicines (properly labelled). If your child gets attacks from contact with cats, pretreat before contact. It is better to start too early than too late. Arrange to call your own doctor for advice if necessary.

Q. How much should a child with asthma drink during an attack?

A. In general, we recommend 50% more than the usual body requirement for size if there is no fever. See General Instructions.

Q. How often are allergy shots given?

A. This can vary considerably. One routine is once or twice a week for the first three to six months, then every one to three weeks.

Q. Do more boys than girls have asthma?

A. Yes, the ratio is about two to one until the teens when the proportion is even.

Q. Why does asthma occur at the most inopportune times?

A. Asthma follows Plaut's Law which states, "If something is going to go wrong, it will be at an inconvenient time." The logic goes as follows: When you are relaxed and well-organized it is possible to keep track of three medications, exposure to cats and ponies, adequate rest and fluid intake. If there is a disruption in your pattern of living because of illness, travelling or the arrival of visitors for the weekend, it is harder to follow the usual routine and to tune into the early signs of an asthma attack.

Q. Where can you buy a peak flow meter?

A. The mini-Wright Peak Flow Meter can be purchased from Armstrong Industries, Chicago, Illinois. Call 800-323-4220 for details.
Information on the Pulmonary Monitor can be obtained from Viltalograph Medical Instruments, Lenexa, Kansas; 800-255-6626.

Q. Does peak flow vary with age?

A. Yes, it varies with age, height and sex.

Q. Sometimes my child benefits a lot from using the inhaler, other times it seems to be of little help; why?

A. Her technique is probably inconsistent. You should check the instructions for inhaler use in Chapter Two.

Q. What is the effect on other children in the family when attention is showered on the child with asthma?

A. Usually not good. Parenting is always a balancing act. It is important to see that everyone in the family receives their share of attention.

Q. What should you do when you sense that your child feels s/he is a nuisance to friends or their families?

A. Plan how to intervene in an asthma attack. Encourage your child to take as much responsibility as possible for the attack. The responsible child is less likely to feel like a nuisance than the helpless child.

Q. Please outline a reasonable plan for treating an asthma attack.

A. - eliminate trigger
    - give medicines
    - give warm liquids
    - limit activity
    - consult doctor if not improving as expected

STAGES IN PARENTS' ABILITY TO MANAGE
AN ASTHMA ATTACK AT HOME

<u>No Knowledge</u>. <u>Responsibility</u>: <u>Parent 0%</u> <u>Physician 100%</u>

Cannot recognize an asthma attack. Knows nothing about medicines.

<u>Beginner</u>. <u>Responsibility</u>: <u>Parent 20%</u> <u>Physician 80%</u>

Can recognize an asthma attack. Needs help in deciding when to start medicine. Cannot judge severity of attack. Cannot communicate clearly with physician on phone.

<u>Intermediate</u>. <u>Responsibility</u>: <u>Parent 40%</u> <u>Physician 60%</u>

Can handle an attack well with doctor's help. Knows how to judge severity of an attack and when to start treatment. Can communicate clearly with physician on phone giving description of progress.

<u>Advanced</u>. <u>Responsibility</u>: <u>Parent 60%</u> <u>Physician 40%</u>

Good knowledge of early clues, triggers and medicines. Skill in monitoring attack and use of medicines. Can handle most attacks at home without consulting physician.

<u>Expert</u>. <u>Responsibility</u>: <u>Parent 80%</u> <u>Physician 20%</u>

Excellent knowledge, skill and attitude. Can handle almost all attacks without consulting physician. Understands the usual course of child's attack and the different types of attack he/she has. Able to analyze course of attacks and make suggestions to physician which improve treatment. Still needs physician for special situations and integration of new medications and treatment at three to twelve month intervals.

Parents should share the responsibility of managing an attack with their physician. Make every office visit an educational experience. The best tool for learning about asthma is the asthma record. Write your observations on it and you will be able to analyze the effects of various triggers and medications.

You should be able to advance to the intermediate state by the time your child has had two attacks. Once you achieve advanced status you will be able to avoid unnecessary hospitalization. Remember, learn something from every office visit and every asthma attack.

I WISH DOCTORS WOULD

Parents in the asthma group completed the sentence, "When dealing with parents of children who have asthma I wish doctors would..." as follows:

-- be as clear and open as possible about all aspects - how to deal with attacks, medication, what's really happening, danger - all the topics dealt with in this workshop

-- tell the parent how long to keep on these high doses of medication before cutting back

-- teach how to prevent attacks

-- I think they do a fine job

-- explain what else goes on besides the wheeze

-- be completely honest--but do not use scare tactics

-- prescribe and stipulate the precise medication but give the boundaries in which I can make decisions on my own

-- have told me sooner that it was asthma I was dealing with instead of a respiratory infection

-- continue just the way they have been

-- assume that the parent is a reasonably intelligent individual who knows her child in a way the doctor doesn't--and that they can learn from each other how to best treat the child

-- explain precautions before an attack and remedies during and after

-- tell us more

-- be straightforward

-- be better informed

-- encourage all concerned to vent their fears

-- make clear the experimental status of the "art"

-- provide lots of information

-- not make me feel that I brought the child in for nothing

-- put articles in newspapers

-- explain everything more

-- if they don't know about asthma--send them to a doctor who knows

Caring for more than 400 families whose children have asthma has taught me that in order to assist parents properly in managing asthma at home I need:

-- the <u>knowledge</u> of the pathophysiology of asthma and the pharmacology of the standard drugs used to treat it

-- the <u>skill</u> to instruct and monitor parents in assessing the severity of asthma, the use of medications and the use of a mini-peak flow meter

-- an <u>attitude</u> which recognizes the parents as the primary managers of their child's asthma

-- the <u>behavior</u> to support them, to be readily accessible, and to treat them as intelligent concerned partners in the care of their child's asthma

Which doctor can help you care for your child with asthma? The physician's specialty is not nearly as important as his/her interest in asthma. Some family practitioners do a better job of caring for children with asthma than do some allergists. An interested pediatrician can take care of about ninety percent of children with asthma without help. S/He will request a consultation from an allergist or a lung specialist to assist in the care of the ten percent of the children who have the most severe or complicated problems. Ideally the pediatrician or family practioner will continue to provide most of the care with occasional consultations from the subspecialist.

<u>Does your child need a consultation</u> with another doctor?

- If your child limits his own activity or misses school because of asthma you should review the situation with your regular doctor or seek a second opinion.

- If your child has to go to the emergency room for care more than once a year her asthma is probably not well controlled. Probably you don't know how to take care of it or it is not being treated adequately. You should review the situation with your doctor or seek another opinion.

- If your physician suggests that your child limit his activities because of asthma it would be wise to seek a second opinion on overall treatment.

What to look for in choosing a doctor:

- Gives written instructions when prescribing medications. This reduces the possibility of misunderstandings and errors in treatment.

- Has his/her staff monitor inhaler use when you come for a visit. Even if they are taught perfectly most people make mistakes and don't get the full benefit of an inhaler unless checked regularly.

- Uses a peak flow meter in the office to assess your child's status. This provides information which is essential for adjusting medications properly.

Please remember, no matter how good the doctor, you have the primary responsibility for your child's care. You live with her and can observe her. The doctor can not. A good doctor will teach you how to care for your child's asthma within certain well-defined limits.

It can be difficult for physicians and patients to make judgments about the management of asthma. Early changes in the bronchioles cannot be felt by the patient or detected by standard means of physical examination. When the patient feels tightness in the chest or starts to wheeze, he is already far into his attack. The stethoscope can detect the problem, but only after the peak expiratory flow rate has dropped by more than 25%. Two new and inexpensive peak flow meters have proved useful in the management of asthma in the doctor's office and at the patient's home.

I use the mini-Wright Peak Flow Meter[1] in the office. It is well calibrated and reliable when used from patient to patient. Since the scale goes down to 60 liters per minute it can be used by a three-year-old. It costs $59.50.

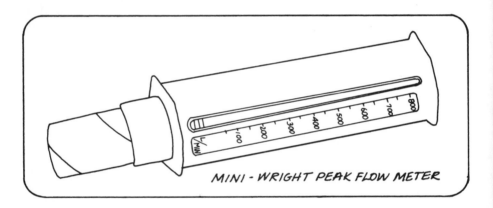

MINI - WRIGHT PEAK FLOW METER

I use it to:
- diagnose asthma
- diagnose exercise-induced asthma
- monitor the patient's progress and to treat an attack in the office
- demonstrate the benefit of an inhaler
- demonstrate to the patient his/her need to take more medicine
- distinguish between asthma and hyperventilation

---

[1]For purchase information call Armstrong Industries Inc., Chicago, Illinois 800-323-4220.

The Pulmonary Monitor[1] costs about $25.00 and, though not as accurate, is adequate for use at home by children who have a peak flow over 150 liters per minute - most six-year-olds.

About 10 percent of my patients use a huffer, either the mini-Wright Peak Flow Meter or the Pulmonary Monitor, at home to:

- show that they are doing okay and do not need to start or change medication
- see if they need more medication (a drop in the huff may indicate the need to increase medication dose). An increase after taking medicine is clear evidence that the medicine was needed.
- check if stable while reducing medication. After a patient has taken several medications for a week or two and the symptoms have cleared s/he may reduce the dose of one medication. If the peak flow rate remains stable s/he can reduce further with less risk of a relapse.
- predict an attack. The peak flow will often drop 24 hours before symptoms of an attack are noticeable. This early warning allows some patients to start medication early - really a big help in the patient whose asthma attacks come on quickly.
- prove that cigarette smoke or other pollutants in the house cause the airways to narrow.
- indicate when to look for triggers of asthma in the environment.
- indicate when to look for early clues of asthma in your body.

To use the mini-Wright Peak Flow Meter or Pulmonary Monitor:

- stand up and move the pointer to zero.
- hold with vent free.
- take in as much air as you can.
- put mouthpiece on tongue and place lips around mouthpiece.
- blow out as hard and fast as possible - a short sharp blast. The meter measures your fastest huff, not your longest.
- huff three times, waiting at least 15 seconds between tries
- record best try morning and night. Try to do this at the same time every day.

---

[1] For purchase information call: Vitalograph Medical Instruments, Lenexa, Kansas 800-255-6626.

What is your normal huff? The huff (maximum peak expiratory flow rate) is related to height and age; it is measured in liters per minute. You can get a rough idea of your normal value by checking a chart of average values. However, there is a great deal of difference between individuals. The best way to find your normal value is to check your huff several times when you are feeling perfectly fine. Consider your best value to be your expected, or normal, value.

What does a change from normal mean? It means that you have a problem and that air is not flowing from your lungs as freely as usual. For example, if you feel fine when you wake up in the morning and get a huff of 350 instead of your usual 400, something is happening. Perhaps you are starting a cold or forgot to take your medicine last night. You could be allergic to your new pillow. It may be that an asthma attack is coming on but the trigger is not evident. Based on past experience you should decide whether to make a change in your medications.

Each person has his own type of types of asthma attack. Some should start taking theophylline and a beta-adrenergic drug by inhaler at the first sign of an attack. Those with milder attacks can often get by with one medication, whereas those with extremely severe attcks may have to use three medicines from the beginning. Some attacks come on very quickly and the huffer can help predict them. Others come on gradually and the huffer can confirm their existence before symptoms are obvious.

Not everyone with asthma will benefit from the home use of a huffer. Some people already understand their attacks, triggers and early warning signs very well. They don't need a huffer. Some children always have clear-cut and ample warning of an attack. They don't need a huffer. Other children and teenagers haven't put all the pieces together. They can benefit from a huffer to confirm their impressions as they learn about their asthma. Many people start out by using the huffer twice daily to get experience with it and to learn about the changes in their flow rate. Later they may use it only with an attack, or once a month to settle a particular question.

Before you start using a huffer at home you should understand enough about asthma to be able to interpret properly the huffer readings. At a minimum you should know the three changes which take place in the bronchioles with an asthma attack and also know how to judge the severity of an attack. The huffer gives you information which can be very helpful if you can put it together with other data.

Problems with technique:

Low reading may be due to poor technique (inadequate effort or slow huff). Since the peak flow rate is the most sensitive measure of lung function available for home use its results should be taken seriously. However using the peak flow meter is not a substitute for understanding how your asthma and your medicines work. It should be a big help but does not tell the whole story.

Comments from Parents and Teenagers:

Emily, age seven: "Uses it when she is having trouble to see how long the effect of the inhaler is lasting. She also uses it when the sitter doesn't know anything about asthma."

Chrystel, age eight: "Very pleased with the huffer. It has helped me detect an oncoming asthma attack before its true onset and I administered her medicine early."

Chuck, age eleven: "Since we live 30 miles from Amherst, we appreciate having a device in the home that is an accurate monitoring device."

Josh, age twelve: "has not bee sick very often lately so we don't use it much, but when he is sick, the huffer is invaluable."

Monica, age fourteen: "I really feel more secure because I know the huffer will tell me to get my butt on medication when I need it."

Bob, age sixteen: "Almost like having a doctor in the house. If I'm doing something wrong like not taking enough medicine, it will show it."

TEACHING MYSELF ABOUT ASTHMA
A Book Review

This book helps parents and children who want to understand the nature of asthma and how to take part in its overall management. It is a Godsend for any practitioner who takes care of children with asthma. Clearly written and well illustrated, it is geared to the reading abilities of children 7 to 12 years of age.

Ideas and facts are presented in a lucid manner. Learning activities are suggested which demonstrate the principles covered. Topics covered include: breathing, pathophysiology, causes, prevention, treatment and the child's role in management.

For several years I have lent copies of this book to parents of every child under my care who has had more than one episode of bronchospactic illness. I suggest that parent and child read the book together before the next visit. Parents are delighted to read material so clearly expressed and easy to understand. The book provides a basis for discussion in future office visits. Because parents understand more clearly the pathophysiology of an asthma attack, its triggers and early warning signs, they are able to intervene earlier and more effectively when an attack occurs. The duration and frequency of office visits is reduced as is the family's dependence on the physician for routine management.

This book, which costs less than an office visit, is a bargain for any family with a child who has asthma.

Teaching Myself About Asthma, by Parcel G., Tiernan K., Nader P., and Weiner L. 147 pages (with 250 illustrations by Mark Weakley).

May be ordered from Health Education Associates, 14 North Lake Road, Columbia, South Carolina 29223. $9.95 prepaid.

adrenalin: adrenergic drug produced by body, same as epinephrine*

albuterol: beta-adrenergic drug*

allergen: any substance that causes the manifestations of allergy

Alupent: a brand name for metaproterenol*

alveolus: air cell of the lungs

antibody: protein which develops in response to an antigen

asymptomatic: without symptoms

asthma: reversible obstructive airway disease

beclomethasone: steroid drug which is taken by inhalation*

bronchi: large windpipes

bronchioles: smaller windpipes

bronchitis: inflammation of the bronchi

bronchodilator: drug which causes the windpipes to open

book: (v.) to leave quickly

cromolyn: type of drug which prevents asthma attacks*

cc: cubic centimeter (1/1000 of a liter), metric measure equal to 1/5 of a measuring teaspoon

decaliter: 1/10 of a liter

---

* See Chapter Three.

dander:	scales of dead skin which may trigger allergy
exacerbation:	worsening
exhale:	breathe out
expiration:	act of breathing out
Gyrocaps:	Slophyllin sustained-release capsule*
hydrocortisone:	steroid drug
IgE:	immunoglobulin gamma E, antibody production of which is often provoked by allergens
inhaler:	device for delivering drug directly into windpipes
inspiration:	act of breathing in
Intal:	a brand name for cromolyn*
intradermal:	into the skin
intravenous:	into the vein
irritant:	substance which bothers
immunotherpay:	desensitization treatment, allergy shots
kg:	kilogram, 1,000 grams or 2.2 pounds
liter:	metric measurement, slightly more than a quart
mean peak flow rate:	highest expiratory rate for age and height expressed in liters per minute
metaproterenol:	adrenergic drug
mg:	milligram, 1/1000 of a gram

* See Chapter Three.

mite:	tiny arachnid found in house dust which may cause allergic asthma
ml:	milliliter, 1/1000 of a liter
mucus:	material produced by glands in windpipes
nebulizer:	equipment for producing fine spray
peak flow rate:	actual highest expiratory flow rate
pollen:	microspores of a seed plant
pollutant:	impurity
prednisone:	steroid drug*
prick test:	skin test for allergy
retraction:	sucking in of the soft tissues in the rib cage
ROAD:	reversible obstructive airway disease
Slophyllin:	a brand name for a theophylline preparation*
Spinhaler:	device for delivering cromolyn sodium*
steroids:	hormones for the adrenal cortex*
sympathomimetic:	produces same effect as stimulation of sympathetic nervous system
Theodur:	a brand name of long-acting theophylline*
theophylline:	generic name of most commonly used bronchodilator*
trigger:	instigator
twitchy:	over-reactive
wheeze:	high-pitched whistling which occurs when air flows through narrowed bronchial tube

* See Chapter Three.

ORDER FORM

You should be able to buy CHILDREN WITH ASTHMA: A MANUAL FOR PARENTS at any bookstore. If this is not possible please use this form.

PEDIPRESS
125 Red Gate Lane
Amherst, MA 01002

Please send _____ copies of CHILDREN WITH ASTHMA: A MANUAL FOR PARENTS @ $9.95 each.

Name: _____

Address: _____

_____Zip: _____

In Massachusetts: please add fifty cents sales tax for each book.

____ I can't wait 3-4 weeks for Book Rate. Here is $2.00 per book for Air Mail.

Send check or money order. No cash or C.O.D.s please.